视觉2020：
中国眼健康报告

―――――――

Vision 2020：
Eye Health in China

全国防盲技术指导组　著
National Committee for the Prevention of Blindness

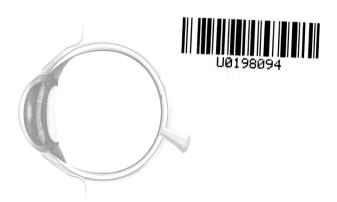

U0198094

人民卫生出版社
·北　京·

图书在版编目（CIP）数据

视觉 2020：中国眼健康报告：汉英对照 / 全国防盲技术指导组著 . —北京：人民卫生出版社，2023.3
ISBN 978-7-117-34622-1

Ⅰ.①视… Ⅱ.①全… Ⅲ.①眼 —保健 —研究报告 —中国 —汉、英 Ⅳ.①R77

中国国家版本馆 CIP 数据核字（2023）第 047041 号

人卫智网	www.ipmph.com	医学教育、学术、考试、健康，购书智慧智能综合服务平台
人卫官网	www.pmph.com	人卫官方资讯发布平台

视觉 2020：中国眼健康报告
Shijue 2020: Zhongguo Yan Jiankang Baogao

著　　者：全国防盲技术指导组
出版发行：人民卫生出版社（中继线 010-59780011）
地　　址：北京市朝阳区潘家园南里 19 号
邮　　编：100021
E - mail：pmph @ pmph.com
购书热线：010-59787592　010-59787584　010-65264830
印　　刷：廊坊一二〇六印刷厂
经　　销：新华书店
开　　本：787 × 1092　1/16　印张：9
字　　数：208 千字
版　　次：2023 年 3 月第 1 版
印　　次：2023 年 4 月第 1 次印刷
标准书号：ISBN 978-7-117-34622-1
定　　价：85.00 元

打击盗版举报电话：010-59787491　E-mail：WQ @ pmph.com
质量问题联系电话：010-59787234　E-mail：zhiliang @ pmph.com
数字融合服务电话：4001118166　E-mail：zengzhi @ pmph.com

《视觉 2020：中国眼健康报告》编委会

Editorial Board of *Vision 2020*: *Eye Health in China*

前　言

　　党和国家历来高度重视人民健康。眼健康是身心健康的重要组成部分,涉及全年龄段人群的全生命周期,包括盲在内的视觉损伤对人民群众的身心健康和生活质量有着严重影响,会加重家庭和社会负担,威胁社会经济生产活动,是涉及民生的重大公共卫生问题和社会问题。我国坚持以人民为中心的发展思想,以提高人民健康水平为核心,在眼健康工作领域,建立并不断完善管理体系、技术指导体系和服务体系。

　　1999年,世界卫生组织联合国际防盲协会发起"视觉2020——享有看见的权利"全球行动倡议,旨在2020年实现消除可避免盲的全球性战略目标,可避免盲包括白内障、沙眼、河盲、儿童盲、屈光不正和低视力等。同年,我国政府作出庄严承诺,并推动相关工作。在"政府主导,各方参与"的工作格局下,我国各级政府大力推进防盲治盲工作,不断完善国家、省(自治区、直辖市)、市级防盲治盲管理体系和县、乡、村眼病防治网络,完善了适合我国国情的眼病防治工作模式,主要致盲性眼病得到有效遏制。针对儿童青少年近视高发问题,我国将近视防控纳入国家战略,实施多部门综合防控,营造了"政府主导、部门配合、专家指导、学校教育、家庭关注"的良好社会氛围。我国活动性沙眼、沙眼性倒睫患病率远低于世界卫生组织确定的致盲性沙眼根治标准,沙眼在我国已经不再是公共卫生问题。我国每百万人白内障手术例数已从1999年的318例提升至2017年的2 205例,增长了近6倍,在"十三五"末期已超过3 000例。白内障患者的手术覆盖率在2014年已经达到62.7%,截至2020年2月,白内障手术覆盖率已超过70%,与既往相比有了大幅度提升。此外,近年来随着我国各地区不断推广适宜技术,急性闭角型青光眼的致盲率已经从20世纪90年代的50%下降到近年来的14.5%,开角型青光眼的检出率则从10%上升到40%。眼科医疗卫生事业快速发展,眼科医务人员参与眼病防治工作的积极性普遍增强。同时,县级医院的眼科服务能力进一步提升,我国约90%的县设有眼科医疗机构,其中约90%可以独立开展白内障复明手术。据2006年与2014年两次九省流调显示,2014年全国50岁以上人群眼盲患病率与2006年相比下降了27%;中、重度视觉损伤患病率与2006年相比下降了16%。

　　随着人口老龄化的加剧、经济社会的快速发展、人民生活方式的改变、社会竞争性压力的增加,年龄相关性眼病、代谢相关性眼病问题凸显,已经成为我国主要的致盲性眼病。此外,由于人均寿命延长、人口总量增加、人口老龄化进程加快,以及人民群众对眼健康需求的不断提高,我国眼病防治工作依然任务艰巨,基层眼保健工作仍需加强,群众爱眼护眼的健康生活理念还需继续强化。

　　2020 年为"视觉 2020——享有看见的权利"行动倡议收官之年,在国家卫生健康委医政医管局的指导下,全国防盲技术指导组编撰发布了《视觉 2020：中国眼健康报告》,旨在全面介绍中国眼健康事业发展的现状,以及在"视觉 2020——享有看见的权利"行动倡议中中国所做的努力与所取得的成果。

王宁利

2020年2月

Foreword

The health of people has always been a priority for the Chinese government. Eye health is an essential component of physical and mental health, concerning the whole life cycle and all age groups. Blindness and visual impairment severely affect people's physical and mental health and quality of life, increase family and social burden, impose a negative impact on social and economic production activities, and thus constitute major public health and social issues. Under the people-centered development principle and with the aim of improving people's health, the government established and has been persistently improving the eye health management system, technical guidance system and service system.

In 1999, the World Health Organization and the International Agency for the Prevention of Blindness jointly launched the "VISION 2020: The Right to Sight" global initiative, with the goal of eliminating avoidable blindness by 2020, including cataract, trachoma, onchocerciasis, childhood blindness, refractive error and low vision. In the same year, the Chinese government made the commitment to promote the initiative and started carrying out relevant work. Under the pattern of "led by government and participated by all parties", governments at all levels vigorously promoted the work of prevention and treatment of blindness and made continuous efforts to improve the national-provincial (autonomous region, municipality directly under the central government)-municipal level management system of prevention and treatment of blindness and county-township-village eye disease prevention and treatment network, thereby developing a working pattern more suited to the reality in China and effectively curbing the leading blinding eye diseases. In view of the high incidence of myopia among children and adolescents, the prevention and treatment of myopia were incorporated into the national strategy, and comprehensive prevention and treatment were implemented through multi-sectoral collaboration, creating a favorable social atmosphere of "leadership by government, cooperation among sectors, guidance by experts, education in school and commitment in family". Currently, the prevalence of active trachoma and trachomatous trichiasis in China is far lower than the elimination threshold set by the WHO and trachoma is no longer a public health issue in China. The cataract surgical rate in China has increased from 318 in 1999 to 2205 in 2017, achieving a 6-fold increase, and is expected to reach about 3000 in 2020. The cataract surgical coverage (CSC) reached 62.7% in 2014, and CSC has been more than 70% by 2020, which has been greatly improved compared with the past. In addition, in recent years, with the nationwide promotion of appropriate techniques, the blindness rate of acute angle-closure glaucoma has decreased from 50% in the 1990s to 14.5% in recent years, and the detection rate of open-angle glaucoma has increased from 10% to 40%. With the rapid advancement in ophthalmic healthcare, the enthusiasm of eye care personnel to participate in the prevention and treatment of eye diseases has been generally boosted. In addition, the eye care service capacity of county-level hospitals has been further improved. At present, about 90% of counties in China have ophthalmic institutions, of which about 90% can provide cataract surgery services independently. According to the survey, in 2014, the prevalence of blindness in the population over 50 years old decreased by 27% compared with 2006, and the prevalence of moderate and severe visual impairment de- creased by 16% compared with 2006.

With population aging, rapid economic and social development, the change of people's life style and the increased pressure due to intense social competition, age-related eye diseases and metabolism-related eye diseases are becoming a prominent issue and the major blinding eye dis- eases in China. What's more, due to the prolongation of life expectancy, the growth of popula- tion, the acceleration of population aging, and enhanced demand for eye health, the prevention and treatment of eye diseases in China remains a challenging task, the eye care service capacity at the primary level still needs to be strengthened, and the eye health awareness should be further improved among the public.

With 2020 being the final year of the VISION 2020 initiative, under the support of the Bu- reau of Medical Administration of the National Health Commission, the National Committee for the Prevention of Blindness developed and launched the *Vision 2020：Eye Health in China*, aim- ing to comprehensively introduce the current eye health situation in China, as well as the efforts and achievements made under the VISION 2020 initiative.

Ningli Wang

2020.2

目 录

第一章 眼健康服务体系 1

 一、政府主导,多方参与,中国眼健康体系逐步完善 1

 二、眼健康规划 2

 三、眼健康政策的转变 3

第二章 中国特色的眼病防治工作模式 5

 一、政府统筹与政策引导 5

 二、学术团体发挥技术优势 6

 三、社会力量积极参与 7

第三章 "视觉 2020"工作进展 10

 一、"视觉 2020"行动倡议 10

 二、中国"视觉 2020"行动 10

 三、消除可避免盲的进展 11

第四章 眼科资源 15

 一、县级眼科机构数量增多、服务能力加强 15

 二、眼科人员队伍不断壮大完善 16

 三、眼科设备配置逐渐完善 18

第五章 盲和视力损伤大幅度下降 20

第六章 主要致盲性眼病疾病谱变化 22

 一、白内障 22

 二、角膜相关疾病 22

 三、黄斑病变、糖尿病视网膜病变等视网膜疾病 23

四、屈光不正 ……………………………………………… 23

五、青光眼 ………………………………………………… 23

六、弱视 …………………………………………………… 24

第七章　近视防控 …………………………………………… 26

一、我国儿童青少年近视的现状 ………………………… 26

二、近视防控的国家战略 ………………………………… 27

三、综合防控措施 ………………………………………… 28

第八章　消灭致盲性沙眼 …………………………………… 30

一、中华人民共和国成立初期，"十人九沙" …………… 30

二、群防群治，科研助力，成效显著 …………………… 30

三、加入"视觉 2020"行动倡议，提前消灭致盲性沙眼 … 31

四、小结 …………………………………………………… 32

第九章　低视力康复 ………………………………………… 34

一、中国低视力康复工作的起步 ………………………… 34

二、低视力康复工作的学术交流 ………………………… 34

三、我国的低视力康复规划 ……………………………… 35

四、我国低视力康复工作取得的成绩 …………………… 35

五、小结 …………………………………………………… 36

第十章　眼健康促进 ………………………………………… 37

一、开展眼健康宣传活动 ………………………………… 37

二、国家大力弘扬眼科医学人文精神 …………………… 38

第十一章　我国眼库发展 …………………………………… 40

一、概况 …………………………………………………… 40

二、我国眼库的现状与问题 ……………………………… 40

三、工作进展 ……………………………………………… 40

第十二章　中国防盲公益活动国际化 ……………………… 42

第十三章　眼科自主研发能力提升 ………………………… 44

一、眼科医疗产品与设备的研发和应用 ………………… 44

二、远程眼科与人工智能的研发与应用 ………………… 45

第十四章　我国眼健康面临的挑战 ·· 48

　　一、屈光不正和白内障疾病负担最重 ····································· 48

　　二、患病率稳中有降,但患病人数上升 ································· 48

　　三、黄斑病变有抬头趋势 ··· 48

　　四、中老年人群疾病负担增长最重 ····································· 49

结束语 ··· 52

致谢 ··· 53

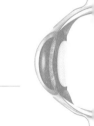

第一章　眼健康服务体系

一、政府主导,多方参与,中国眼健康体系逐步完善

中国政府高度重视防盲治盲事业,自"全国防盲和眼保健'七五'规划(1988—1990年)"以来,每五年制定防盲治盲或眼健康规划,规划中不断强化政府责任,完善三级防盲治盲网络,加强防盲治盲队伍建设,持续改善和提高基层眼健康服务能力[1]。

近年来,国家颁布一系列关于推进医疗联合体建设和发展、推进分级诊疗制度建设、全面提升县级医院综合诊疗能力的政策。政府也随之在眼健康领域制定了相应政策[2],如鼓励城市三级医院眼科、眼科医院与县级综合医院眼科、基层医疗卫生机构建立协作体,成立全国眼科联盟,开展形式多样的纵向合作,提升眼科诊疗和眼健康服务整体水平;加强眼科医疗机构与疾病预防控制机构或眼病防治机构、低视力康复机构的沟通协作,建立医、防、康复相结合的合作机制;以县级公立医院综合改革和三级医院对口帮扶贫困县县医院等工作为契机,大力推动县域眼科医疗服务能力建设;完善初级眼保健服务纳入初级卫生保健体系,加强基层特别是农村地区眼病防治工作,探索建立基层眼病防治工作模式。

1984 年 12 月 6 日,我国成立全国防盲技术指导组。全国防盲技术指导组是由具有防盲治盲经验和业务指导能力的专业人员组成,以开展全国防盲工作为目的的专业性组织。其主要职责为在国家卫生健康委领导下,制定全国防盲治盲规划,协助国家卫生健康委和各级卫生健康行政部门,落实全国防盲治盲规划,组织防盲治盲专业人员培训,研究推广适宜眼科技术,开展防盲治盲相关学术交流等。全国防盲技术指导组成立后,立即着手全国防盲流行病调查、县级防盲工作者教材编写与培训,开展了创建防盲先进县示范工程,组织各省(自治区、直辖市)、市成立防盲技术指导组,建立国家、省(自治区、直辖市)、市和县、乡、村两个眼病防治工作网络。防盲网络的构建使我国眼健康的工作能够上传下达,提高了眼健康工作组织的协同性与实施效率,充分发挥各级机构的积极性、主动性和创造性,群策群力,汇集了广大眼科医务人员和社会各界力量,保证了国家的防盲政策能够在基层及时贯彻和落实,切实提高和加强了基层人民群众对眼健康的认识,做到国家眼健康政策普惠大众。

中国残疾人联合会在眼健康服务方面也开展了相关工作,致力于开展盲和低视力的流行病学调查、预防、康复及专业人才的培养,组织专家和学术团体举办国际低视力康复论坛,开展低视力康复骨干人才培训。

二、眼健康规划

长期以来,国家卫生行政部门制定全国防盲和眼健康规划,用于指导全国各省开展防盲工作。"全国防盲和眼保健'七五'规划(1988—1990年)"是首个防盲和眼保健规划,包括防盲奋斗目标、主要任务、开展试点、保障措施等方面,在卫生保健计划中强调人员培养、卫生保健服务能力、学校眼病防治计划的制定;在初级眼卫生保健计划中包含了编写教材、举办培训班、培训基层卫生人员、收集盲和低视力资料、健康宣教和建立有效转诊制度等;在其他工作中强调建立信息监测系统,健全登记报告、资料收集制度,逐步形成网络,重点收集试点区的防盲情况,在全国统一标准的流行病学基础上开展普治工作,统一组织适当规模的眼科医疗队帮助试点区治疗白内障,并实行专业机构和当地初级眼保健人员相结合,不断提高手术率,使经治盲人达到现有可治盲人的60%。建立健全研究系统,有条件的省建立科研中心(所),重点解决防盲亟需解决的技术问题,充分体现当时的时代特色[3]。

1992年,卫生部下发《关于1991—2000年全国防盲和初级眼保健工作规划的通知》(卫医发〔1992〕1号),该规划基于中国支持世界卫生组织(World Health Organization,WHO)提出的"2000年人人享有卫生保健"全球性战略目标而制定。在工作措施中较前一次规划更完善,主要从加强全国及各省(自治区、直辖市)、市防盲技术指导组的建设,建立防盲队伍、培养专业人员、将初级眼保健纳入初级卫生保健,继续发展和巩固防盲治盲先进县,预防常见眼病、减少新发盲人,加强防盲治盲科学研究、在初级眼保健工作规范化等方面做了相关规划与要求[4]。

2006年,为了进一步推进我国防盲治盲工作,为最终实现到2020年消除可避免盲的战略目标奠定坚实基础,保障人民群众身体健康,促进经济社会协调发展,国家印发了《全国防盲治盲规划(2006—2010年)》(卫医发〔2006〕282号)。规划提出要加强领导、健全组织机构、整合社会资源,加强防盲治盲队伍和基层防盲治盲工作能力的建设,创建防盲治盲示范县(区)和白内障无障碍县(区),加强对贫困视力残疾人的医疗救助和康复工作,做好防盲治盲的宣传教育工作,加强防盲治盲的调查研究,建立防盲信息系统[5]。

2012年,卫生部、中国残联印发的《全国防盲治盲规划(2012—2015年)》(卫医政发〔2012〕52号)中提出,中国人口基数大,盲和低视力损伤的患者仍有很多,存在眼科医疗资源总量不足、分布不均和质量不高,基层眼保健工作薄弱、信息系统不完善等问题。因此,在此次规划中提出进一步建立完善防盲治盲工作网,加强防盲治盲人员队伍建设,防治主要致盲性眼病,开展低视力康复工作,开展防盲治盲宣传教育工作,制定基层常见致盲性眼病防治工作指南,进一步完善白内障复明手术信息报送制度七个方面的内容[6]。

2016年,国家卫生计生委印发了《"十三五"全国眼健康规划(2016—2020年)》(国卫医发〔2016〕57号)。规划名称由防盲治盲规划改为眼健康规划,把我国的防盲治盲工作推上一个新台阶。规划提出,要把眼病防治工作纳入各级政府卫生事业发展规划和健康扶贫工作计划,加强与残联、教育、民政、财政等部门的沟通协调。规划明确了七方面的工作措施,包括完善眼病防治服务体系;加强人员队伍建设,推动可持续发展;防治导致盲和视觉损伤的主要眼病;规范开展低视力康复工作;开展眼健康宣传教育工作;加强数据收集与信息化建设;完善政府主导、多方协作的工作机制[1]。

三、眼健康政策的转变

自"七五"规划至今,中国政府一直为眼健康工作创建积极的政策环境。在党和政府的高度重视下,经过多方面的共同努力,我国主要致盲性眼病已由沙眼为主的传染性疾病转变为代谢性、慢性、年龄相关性眼病。儿童青少年近视、高度近视性眼底病变、糖尿病视网膜病变、老年性黄斑病变等眼病日益成为需要关注的重点,国家政策也与时俱进,防盲工作的重点也从防盲治盲向眼健康管理、眼病的预防转变[2],并由最初的防盲治盲规划转变为眼健康规划。

由于80%的致盲性眼病是可防可控的[7],这些疾病多需要早发现并进行合理适时干预,因此,防盲工作模式由单一的防盲治盲转变为多方面的眼健康管理,当前更注重的是将关口前移,资源下沉,将初级眼保健纳入初级卫生保健中,将眼科疾病纳入慢性病管理,建立眼健康档案,眼保健追踪随访等长效化机制。防盲项目由"输血"模式转变为"造血"模式,方式由帮扶、免费救治向教育培训转移;过去的防盲项目多为流动项目,近些年逐渐转变为"中国县级医院眼科团队培训"等,为当地培养专业人才,增强基层的软实力,使技术和人才在当地生根,逐步形成可持续发展的模式。

参 考 文 献

1. 中华人民共和国国家卫生和计划生育委员会. 国家卫生计生委关于印发"十三五"全国眼健康规划 (2016—2020 年) 的通知 (国卫医发〔2016〕57 号)[EB/OL].(2016-11-09)[2020-04-12]. www. nhc. gov. cn/ zwgk/zxgzjh/201611/9463afb00ac84910bb3c22f8629cf90a. shtml.
2. 中华人民共和国国家卫生和计划生育委员会, 中华人民共和国国家中医药管理局. 关于进一步做好分级诊疗制度建设有关重点工作的通知 (国卫医发〔2018〕28 号)[EB/OL].(2018-08-07)[2020-04-12]. http:// www. nhc. gov. cn/xxgk/pages/viewdocument. jsp？dispatchDate=&staticUrl=/yzygj/s3594q/201808/1c4adec 50bfb4bf9b0803a5940b8bf14. shtml.
3. 中华人民共和国卫生部. 关于下发《全国防盲计划大纲》和《全国防盲和眼保健七五规划》的通知 [EB/ OL].(1988-07-14)[2020-04-13]. http://www. moheyes. com/News/Details/9854fdd1-b63b-4254-b4f6- f51b2bc210ab.
4. 《中国卫生年鉴》编辑委员会. 中国卫生年鉴: 1993 年 [M]. 北京: 人民卫生出版社, 1993: 181.
5. 中华人民共和国卫生部. 关于印发《全国防盲治盲规划 (2006~2010 年)》的通知 (卫医发〔2006〕282号) [EB/OL].(2006-07-26)[2020-04-13]. http://www. nhc. gov. cn/wjw/gfxwj/201304/e6a33b8930ba445da6988ca 012562d75. shtml.

6. 中华人民共和国卫生部, 中国残联. 关于印发全国防盲治盲规划 (2012-2015 年) 的通知 (卫医政发〔 2012 〕52 号)[EB/OL].(2012-07-27)[2020-04-13]. http://www. nhc. gov. cn/jnr/qgayrbmgz/201406/29f041a9126c484e87b8e7c36dc91b24. shtml.

7. World Health Organization. 普遍的眼健康: 2014-2019 年全球行动计划.[EB/OL].(2013-05-24)[2020-04-19]. https://apps. who. int/iris/bitstream/handle/10665/105937/9789245506560_chi. pdf; jsessionid=938CF4336F6ED37306821D82CE8076BB ? sequence=9.

第二章 中国特色的眼病防治工作模式

中国防盲工作坚持以政府为主导,多部门协作、全社会参与的眼病防治工作模式,为人民群众提供全面、公平、可及的眼健康服务。

一、政府统筹与政策引导

健康中国建设,是全面建成小康社会、基本实现社会主义现代化的重要基础,是全面提升中华民族健康素质、实现人民健康与经济社会协调发展的国家战略,是积极参与全球健康治理、履行 2030 年可持续发展议程国际承诺的重大举措[1]。眼健康是国民健康的重要组成部分,因而需要不断推进我国眼健康事业发展,以进一步提高人民群众的眼健康水平[2]。

截至 2019 年末,我国全口径基本医疗保险参保人数为 135 436 万人,参保覆盖面稳定在 95% 以上,基本实现人员全覆盖[3]。2020 年,白内障被纳入农村贫困人口大病专项救治病种[4]。此外,为了进一步提高医疗可负担性,实现大众医疗均等化,政府采取了多项具体医疗改革措施。例如,开展日间手术,减少患者住院时间、等待时间、降低医疗费用,充分利用医院床位[5]。随着药品“零加成”政策在公立医院全面推开,进行零差率销售,给患者真正带来了实惠,避免了“因病返贫”的现象[6]。

2016 年国家卫生计生委印发《“十三五”全国眼健康规划(2016—2020 年)》(国卫医发〔2016〕57 号),明确各级眼科专科医院、综合医院眼科、设有眼科的妇幼保健机构和基层医疗卫生机构的职责、任务和要求,提供全面、公平、可及的眼科医疗服务。充分发挥国家级、省级防盲技术指导组和眼科专业学会和协会的专业优势,组织开展基层眼科及相关卫生技术人员的培训,提高常见眼病诊治能力,发挥其作为基层眼科医疗服务指导中心的作用,从而进一步落实分级诊疗[2]。鉴于我国城乡资源差异大,作为基层防盲治盲工作的主要实施者,县级医院存在着眼健康工作薄弱、人才缺乏等问题,2016 年 5 月 18 日,全国防盲技术指导组牵头启动了中国县级医院眼科团队培训项目,旨在为县级医院培养可独立提供高质量眼科服务的团队,同时以三级培训模式为基础,建立我国基层眼健康服务能力建设标准化培训模式,截至 2019 年年底,项目培训县级医院 70 余家,培训县级眼科团队人员约 350 名,培训乡医 3 070 人,培训教师 1 686 人,成人白内障筛查 487 308 人,儿童屈光不正筛查 328 317 人。

二、学术团体发挥技术优势

儿童青少年近视是引起全社会共同关注的重要问题。2018 年 8 月,习近平总书记作出重要指示,强调全社会都要行动起来,共同呵护好孩子的眼睛,让他们拥有一个光明的未来。为了进一步做好近视防治工作,教育部、国家卫生健康委等部委联合印发了《综合防控儿童青少年近视实施方案》(教体艺〔2018〕3 号)[7]。为了落实指示、批示,更好地开展工作,同时充分发挥全国防盲技术指导组、眼科专家和眼科医疗机构在眼健康方面的指导作用,全国防盲技术指导组成立了近视防治专家组,为国家和各级卫生健康部门提供有关近视防治的专业技术建议,为医疗机构和眼科医务人员科学规范地矫正近视提供指导,为近视防治相关流行病学调查研究的开展提供帮助。此外,受国家卫生健康委委托,全国防盲技术指导组组织专家编写了《近视防治指南》《斜视诊治指南》和《弱视诊治指南》[8]。

中国是全球 2 型糖尿病患者最多的国家,随着糖尿病患者的增多,糖尿病视网膜病变的患病率、致盲率也逐年升高,是目前工作年龄人群第一位的致盲性疾病。循证医学研究证明,严格控制血糖、血脂、血压等多种危险因素,同时进行眼底筛查,可显著降低糖尿病患者发生糖尿病视网膜病变的危险性;对早期糖尿病视网膜病变患者采取有效的干预措施,则可显著降低糖尿病视网膜病变致盲率。目前,87% 的糖尿病患者就诊于县级及以下医疗机构,但是糖尿病视网膜病变的基本诊疗措施和适宜技术却在三级医疗机构实施[9]。因此,全国防盲技术指导组组织专家编写了《中国糖尿病视网膜病变防治指南(基层版)》和《糖尿病视网膜病变分级诊疗服务技术方案》[9,10],以分级诊疗制度为基础,进一步提高基层规范化治疗水平,建立早期筛查、诊断、转诊与治疗的有效模式,降低群众的疾病负担[10]。

2017 年 9 月 9 日,在全国防盲技术指导组牵头下,共有 146 家医院参与的全国眼科联盟正式成立。该联盟的成立旨在集中全国眼科学专业力量,充分利用互联网等前沿技术,实现专家、临床、科研、教学、患者等各种资源的共享,以患者为中心,执行分级诊疗和逐级转诊制度;同时通过加强眼科医师规范化培训和眼科人才培养,带动提升全国眼科人才整体素质。此外,全国眼科联盟还建立了科研平台,推动临床科研发展和成果转化,引领我国眼科医学研究方向,提高全国眼科医学研究水平,实现多中心临床数据与病例资源在成员单位间共享,通过大数据分析,系统了解我国国民眼健康现状,从而为国家制定防盲治盲政策提供依据。全国多中心青光眼研究联盟"青光眼百家联盟"于 2014 年正式成立,旨在进一步深入开展青光眼遗传学研究,搭建科研平台,开展高质量的多中心临床研究,培养临床研究人员,提高临床科研能力,并通过联盟推广新技术、新项目。为了进一步推动各级医院的青光眼诊疗水平、有效贯彻青光眼学组诊疗指南和规范,联盟建立了自己的临床试验电子数据采集系统(Electric Data Capture,EDC),实现了对数据的有效质量控制。中华医学会眼科学分会每年举办全国眼科年会,除了在全体大会上的防盲专题报告,还专门设立防盲专场,讨论防盲领域的新观念、新进展、新技术及新理念。针对我国常见致盲性眼病,中华医学会眼科学分会各专业学组陆续发布了多个专家共识或指南,如青光眼学组发布了《我国原发性青光眼诊断和治疗专家共识》;眼底病学组发布了《我国糖尿病视网膜病变临床诊疗指南》;角膜病学组发布了《感染性角膜病临床诊疗专家共识》;眼视光学组发布了《重视高度近视防控的专家共识》;白内障学组发布了《我国白内障术后急性细菌性眼内炎治疗专家共识》;斜视与小儿眼科学组发布了《弱视诊断专家共识》等。这些专家共识和指南的发布规范了我国常见致盲性眼病的诊疗,有助于降低我国常见致盲性眼病的致盲率。

"预防为主"是新中国成立后三次卫生工作方针中唯一没有改变的内容。大部分眼病属于慢性病,且其中80%的致盲性眼病是可防可控的[11],只有重视眼病的防控才能缓解大医院人满为患的局面。在"十三五"规划期间,我国眼健康工作重点从"防盲治盲"转变为"眼健康服务",强调从眼健康的影响因素入手实施干预,坚持预防为主、关口前移[2]。中华预防医学会公共卫生眼科学分会是国内首个正式成立的将公共卫生与眼病防治结合在一起的专业性组织,旨在促进我国公共卫生眼科事业的发展,提高眼科公共卫生和预防医学学科的水平,有效提高眼科疾病的防控能力。该分会的成立加强了眼科与公共卫生的结合,每年举办以教育基层医生为主的培训班,为基层培养具有公共卫生眼科思维的医生。此外,分会也不定期举办聚焦公共卫生眼科热点、焦点的高水平学术会议和学术论坛。在新冠肺炎疫情期间,中华预防医学会公共卫生眼科学分会委员们以国家发布的指南性文件为基础,从预防医学和眼科学角度,提出眼科防护建议,为眼科临床工作应该采取的防护措施提供全面、细致、实用的建议,发表了《新型冠状病毒疫情期间眼科防护专家建议》中、英文版,并且还出版了《新型冠状病毒肺炎眼科防护手册》,为共同抗击疫情贡献力量。

三、社会力量积极参与

目前,公立医院仍然是国内眼科医疗服务的主要承担者,但是近年来,在促进社会办医的一系列医改政策的支持下,社会资本广泛进入医疗卫生领域,社会办医已成为我国医疗资源的重要组成部分。民营眼科医院的成立一方面弥补了眼科医疗卫生资源的不足,另一方面利用优质民营眼科医院的灵活性,引入了先进的眼科医院管理模式和服务体系。截至2018年,我国医疗卫生机构眼科床位数已达到13万,年门急诊量为1.2亿[12],根据有关调查报告,民营眼科卫生医疗机构的市场规模占全国眼科服务市场的五分之一。此外,随着生活水平的提高,人们对眼健康管理、特色眼科服务等中高端眼科医疗的需求日益增长,形成了多层次、多样化的眼科医疗服务需求态势,民营眼科的发展可以提升眼科医疗服务资源的整体利用效率并满足城乡居民多层次的眼科医疗服务需求。

随着我国眼健康工作的推进,许多非政府组织积极参与到了中国的防盲工作中。1997年,国家卫生行政部门与国际狮子会共同启动了"视觉第一中国行动"。该项目自启动以来,已实施了三期:项目一期和二期共组派了548批医疗队,开展了503万例白内障复明手术,援建了210个县医院眼科,建立了6个区域培训中心和25个省级培训基地,培训了6万余名眼科卫生技术人员;项目三期开展"2016年前在中国根治致盲性沙眼"项目,进行沙眼的评估、筛查和治疗[13]。

1997年,中华健康快车基金会成立,到2019年底,"健康快车"或者医院行遍全国28个省(自治区、直辖市)的121个地区,停靠187个服务站点,为21万余名贫困白内障患者实施了复明手术。"糖尿病视网膜病变筛查"项目在全国21个省(自治区、直辖市)建立了40家糖尿病视网膜病变筛查中心,帮助235名医生获得国际认证的糖网阅片师资质证书,累计筛查糖尿病患者19万余人,其中筛查出濒临失明的糖尿病患者6 700多名。

国际奥比斯组织从1982年起在中国展开防盲工作,30余年共完成41次飞机医院项目。在32个省(自治区、直辖市)开展230个项目。培训卫生工作者70 000人次,受益人数超过1 700万。

弗雷德·霍洛基金会1998年起着手在中国开展消除可避免盲的工作。20余年来,该基金会的中国项目培训卫生工作者超过30 000人次,为近300万人进行了视力筛查,还为140余万眼病患者提供了手术和治疗。

"亮睛工程"于2004年在香港发起,旨在中国发展可持续的防盲复明工程。截至2018年10月,"亮睛工程"共在全国10个省级行政区设立了30个扶贫眼科中心,完成163 839例白内障复明手术,培训超过140名白内障手术医生。

亚洲防盲基金会一直致力于为亚洲发展中国家开展防盲治盲项目,并于1995年设立中国复明扶贫流动眼科手术车项目,截至2019年,已帮助逾64万名贫困白内障患者成功复明。

参 考 文 献

1. 中华人民共和国中共中央国务院."健康中国2030"规划纲要.[EB/OL].(2016-10-25)[2020-04-05]. http://www. gov. cn/xinwen/2016-10/25/content_5124174. htm.
2. 中华人民共和国国家卫生和计划生育委员会. 国家卫生计生委关于印发"十三五"全国眼健康规划(2016—2020年)的通知(国卫医发〔2016〕57号)[EB/OL].(2016-11-09)[2020-04-05]. www. nhc. gov. cn/zwgk/zxgzjh/201611/9463afb00ac84910bb3c22f8629cf90a. shtml
3. 中华人民共和国国家医疗保障局.2019年医疗保障事业发展统计快报.[EB/OL].(2020-03-30)[2020-04-05]. http://www. nhsa. gov. cn/art/2020/3/30/art_7_2930. html.
4. 中华人民共和国国家卫生健康委员会, 中华人民共和国民政部, 中华人民共和国国务院扶贫办综合司, 等.关于进一步扩大农村贫困人口大病专项救治病种范围的通知.(国卫办医发〔2020〕338号)[EB/OL].(2020-04-26)[2021-07-14]. http://www. gov. cn/zhengce/zhengceku/2020-04/28/content_5507149. htm.
5. 史力群,夏仲方,潘云龙.推进日间手术规范化管理的思考[J].现代医学,2015,15(11):9-10.
6. 徐君花.浅谈公立医院药品零差价的影响及措施[J].现代经济信息,2014,(10):316-325.
7. 中华人民共和国教育部, 中华人民共和国国家卫生健康委员会, 中华人民共和国国家体育总局, 等.教育部等八部门关于印发《综合防控儿童青少年近视实施方案》(教体艺〔2018〕3号)的通知.[EB/OL].(2018-04-05)[2020-08-30]. http://www. moe. gov. cn/srcsite/A17/moe_943/s3285/201808/t20180830_346672. html.
8. 中华人民共和国国家卫生健康委员会.关于印发《近视防治指南、斜视诊治指南和弱视诊治指南》(国卫办医函〔2018〕393号)的通知.[EB/OL].(2018-06-01)[2020-04-05]. http://www. moe. gov. cn/jyb_xwfb/xw_zt/moe_357/jyzt_2019n/2019_zt7/zcjj/bw/201904/t20190428_379876. html
9. 中华人民共和国国家卫生健康委员会. 国家卫生计生委办公厅关于印发糖尿病视网膜病变分级诊疗服

务技术方案的通知.(国卫办医函〔2017〕280 号)[EB/OL].(2017-04-01)[2020-04-05]. http://www. nhc. gov. cn/ yzygj/s7653/201704/3524f29f1599419aa04bbe4e068c962a. shtml.

10. 全国防盲技术指导组. 中国糖尿病视网膜病变防治指南 (基层版)[M]. 北京: 人民卫生出版社. 2017: 2

11. World Health Organization. 普遍的眼健康: 2014-2019 年全球行动计划.[EB/OL].(2013-05-24)[2020-04-19]. https://apps. who. int/iris/bitstream/handle/10665/105937/9789245506560_chi. pdf; jsessionid=938CF 4336F6ED37306821D82CE8076BB? sequence=9.

12. 国家卫生健康委员会. 2019 中国卫生健康统计年鉴.[M]. 北京: 中国协和医科大学出版社. 2020: 81, 122

13. 王宁利, 胡爱莲, Hugh R Taylor. 沙眼 [M]. 北京: 人民卫生出版社 2015: 39.

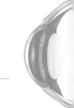

第三章 "视觉 2020" 工作进展

一、"视觉 2020" 行动倡议

"视觉 2020" 行动倡议是由 WHO 联合国际防盲协会(International Agency for the Prevention of Blindness, IAPB)于 1999 年 2 月 18 日发起的全球性行动。"视觉 2020" 行动倡议的目标是至 2020 年在全球范围内消除可避免盲,逆转可避免视觉损伤在 1990—2020 年间翻倍的这一趋势。"视觉 2020" 行动倡议旨在提高关键人群对于可避免盲的主要致盲原因及解决办法的认知度;开发并保证防盲治盲活动所必需的资源;在世界各国推动 "视觉 2020" 国家级项目的规划、制定与实施。与初级卫生保健相结合的疾病控制、人力资源发展、基础设施建设及适宜技术应用是 "视觉 2020" 的三大核心战略[1-2]。

2006 年,世界卫生大会(World Health Assembly, WHA)通过了 WHA59.25 号决议,在 2003 年 WHA56.26 号决议根治可避免盲的基础之上,提出将预防可避免视觉损伤也纳入了 "视觉 2020" 工作重点。

2013 年 WHA 上,66.4 号决议《普遍的眼健康:2014—2019 全球行动计划》通过,虽然该决议是作为 "视觉 2020" 行动倡议的一部分,但是将目标调整为到 2019 年将可避免视觉损伤的患病率降低 25%(与 2010 年的基线患病率相比),与原本的 2020 年前实现全球消除可避免视觉损伤的目标相比,该目标的可实现性更高[3]。该决议最终目标是减少可成为全球公共卫生问题的可避免视觉损伤,保证已经发生视觉损伤的人接受康复服务[4]。

二、中国 "视觉 2020" 行动

1999 年 9 月,"视觉 2020" 行动倡议正式在西太平洋区域启动,我国是西太平洋地区第一个启动 "视觉 2020" 行动倡议的国家。时任卫生部部长张文康在北京代表我国政府在宣言上签字,庄严承诺:2020 年以前,我国消除可避免盲。可避免盲包括白内障、沙眼、河盲、儿童盲、低视力与屈光不正,其中河盲只存在于某些非洲及少数拉美国家,在我国不存在[4]。2006 年,国家印发了《全国防盲治盲规划(2006—2010 年)》(卫医发〔2006〕282 号)。到

2008 年底,全国有 27 个省(自治区、直辖市)已经制定了防盲治盲 5 年规划或草案[5]。2012 年,国家在"十一五"期间取得的工作进展之上,结合"视觉 2020"行动倡议核心战略,印发了《全国防盲治盲规划(2012—2015 年)》(卫医政发〔2012〕52 号)。2016 年,国家根据健康中国建设、深化医药卫生体制改革工作总体要求以及 WHO《普遍的眼健康:2014—2019 全球行动计划》决议,为继续推进我国"十三五"期间眼健康事业,进一步提高人民群众的眼健康水平,制定了《"十三五"全国眼健康规划(2016—2020 年)》(国卫医发〔2016〕57 号)。

我国以实施该行动为契机,将防治可避免视觉损伤的工作整合到国家健康计划和健康服务的供给中,将眼科医疗服务纳入医疗服务体系的整体中发展,继续完善农村防盲治盲网络,开展眼科医疗资源和眼病流行病学调查,加大防盲治盲宣传教育力度,使防盲治盲工作不再局限于防治眼病的范围[6,7]。此外,通过建立并不断完善国家和省、市级防盲治盲管理体系、技术指导体系和服务体系,充分调动防盲资源,构建了"政府主导、各方参与"的工作格局[8]。为了提高关键人群对于可避免盲的主要致盲原因及解决办法的认知度,每年 6 月6 日在全国范围内举办以可避免盲防治为主题的"爱眼日"宣传活动[9]。人力资源发展、基础设施建设方面,我国也取得了显著进展。我国可提供眼科医疗服务的县级医院的数量和设有独立眼科的县级医院数量分别从 2003 年的 1 995 所和 1 033 所[10]增加至 2018 年的3 478 所和 1 807 所;眼科医师也由 2003 年的 1.91 万人[10]发展到 2018 年的 4.48 万人。在适宜技术推广方面,针对主要致盲性眼病,出台《儿童眼及视力保健技术规范》《儿童青少年近视防控适宜技术指南》《早产儿治疗用氧和视网膜病变防治指南》等多个规范与指南,通过眼病防治工作网络推广主要眼病的适宜防治技术,提升各级网络眼病防治服务能力,特别是基层和农村地区的眼病防治工作能力。

三、消除可避免盲的进展

"视觉 2020"行动倡议的目标为消除包括白内障、沙眼、河盲、儿童盲及低视力与屈光不正等导致的可避免盲,我国没有河盲。

白内障是我国的首位致盲性眼病,每百万人白内障手术例数(cataract surgery rate,CSR)是 WHO《普遍的眼健康:2014—2019 全球行动计划》三大监测指标之一[11]。我国经过开展白内障免费救治项目、实现医保逐步全覆盖、提升县级医疗机构眼科服务水平等全方位的长期努力,CSR 已从 1999 年的 318[12]提升至 2017 年的 2 205,提前实现了《"十三五"全国眼健康规划》提出的我国 CSR 要在 2020 年年底达到 2 000 以上的目标(图 3-1)。

除白内障外,沙眼也是"视觉 2020"行动倡议关注的眼病。20 世纪 40 至 50 年代,沙眼是我国的首位致盲眼病。1987 年我国沙眼致残率占各种视力残疾的 14.25%,已由首位降为第三位;2006 年我国沙眼致残率减为 1.87%,沙眼已不再是主要致盲性眼病。2014 年底评估结果显示:在 1~9 岁儿童中活动性沙眼低于 5%,成年人中沙眼倒睫低于 0.1%,达到了WHO 提出的消灭致盲性沙眼的目标[13]。2015 年,在瑞士举行的 WHA 上,国家卫生计生委主任李斌同志在一般性辩论发言中正式宣布:我国已在 2014 年达到了 WHO 根治致盲性沙眼的要求。这意味着我国已提前实现消灭致盲性沙眼的目标。2019 年,WHO 按照新的流

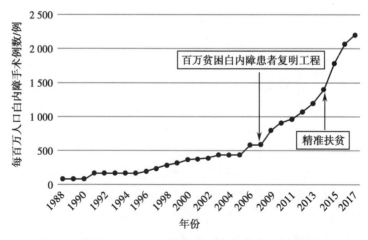

图 3-1 我国 1998—2017 年每百万人白内障手术例数变化

程和标准对我国消灭致盲性沙眼工作进行了认证。

儿童盲占盲人总数的比例较低,但由于儿童处于生命周期早期,伤残调整寿命年数和残疾时间长,儿童盲往往会给家庭和社会带来巨大负担。研究表明,有 1/3 到 1/2 的儿童盲是可避免或者可治疗的[14]。导致儿童视力发育异常甚至盲或低视力的眼病包括:早产儿视网膜病变、先天性白内障、先天性青光眼、新生儿淋菌性结膜炎、弱视、斜视、高度屈光不正、屈光参差、先天性上睑下垂、视网膜母细胞瘤等。多年来,我国政府一直积极推进儿童盲的早筛早治工作,其中,北京早产儿视网膜病变发病率已经从 20 世纪 90 年代的 20.3% 降至 2005 年的 10.8%,致盲率大幅度下降[15]。2004 年,《早产儿治疗用氧和视网膜病变防治指南》[16]发布以后,在北京、上海、广州、深圳等地基本上形成了由一家眼科中心负责,多家新生儿重症监护病房联合的筛查体系。

2006 年第二次全国残疾人抽样调查显示,0~6 岁儿童筛查的 51 328 人中,视力残疾共 193 例,视力残疾率为 3.76‰,其中遗传、先天异常或发育障碍 93 例,视力残疾率为 1.8‰,弱视致视力残疾共 61 例,视力残疾率为 1.18‰,屈光不正 19 例,视力残疾率为 0.37‰。2013 年,为了提高儿童保健工作质量,进一步规范相关领域儿童保健服务的内容、方法、流程和考核评估,国家印发《关于印发儿童眼及视力保健等儿童保健相关技术规范的通知》(卫办妇社发〔2013〕26 号)。2019 年,国家发布《关于做好 0~6 岁儿童眼保健和视力检查有关工作的通知》(国卫办妇幼发〔2019〕9 号),要求加快建立和完善居民电子健康档案信息系统,尽快实现 0~6 岁儿童视力健康档案电子化管理,确保 0~6 岁儿童健康档案中儿童视力健康档案相关内容在儿童入学时完整、准确、顺利提取,并及时移交教育机构。此外,在《七岁以下儿童保健和健康情况年报表》中新增 "0~6 岁儿童眼保健和视力检查人数" "6 岁儿童视力检查人数" "6 岁儿童视力不良检出人数" 等统计指标。承担基本公共卫生服务的医疗卫生机构要对辖区内每年开展 0~6 岁儿童眼保健和视力检查工作情况进行统计。此外,将 0~6 岁儿童眼保健和视力检查覆盖率及视力健康电子档案建立情况已纳入考核体系,要求自 2019 年起,0~6 岁儿童每年眼保健和视力检查覆盖率达 90% 以上。

1991 年,我国将低视力康复工作纳入《中国残疾人事业 "八五" 计划纲要(1991 年—

1995 年)》。中国残疾人联合会(以下简称"中国残联")将低视力康复工作作为重点工作之一,通过设立低视力康复部、培训人员、开发供应助视器具、宣传普及知识等措施,已为数十万名低视力者配用助视器;通过出版低视力专著《临床低视力学》和全国高等教材《低视力学》以及各级各类培训班,培训了大量的低视力康复专业人员、儿童低视力家长等。《"十三五"全国眼健康规划(2016—2020 年)》(国卫医发〔2016〕57 号)中明确指出:三级综合医院眼科和眼科专科医院应普遍提供低视力门诊服务,有条件的医院要开展低视力康复工作。建立眼科医疗机构与低视力康复机构的合作、转诊工作机制。加强低视力人才队伍建设,推动可持续发展[9]。同时,国家财政加大投入支持助视器专业验配及康复培训,并且大力支持具有自主产权的助视器的研发。

屈光不正中的近视是世界范围内发病率最高且年龄跨度最大的眼健康问题,其中高度近视视网膜病变在致盲原因中占相当高的比例,未矫正屈光不正的防治已成为我国眼健康工作的重要内容,相关近视防控已成为我国国家战略。八部委制定了《综合防控儿童青少年近视实施方案》(教体艺〔2018〕3 号)等相关政策,并印发了一系列技术指南、防控手册等。各地相继展开儿童青少年近视率基数调查,组织专家们对各地近视调查工作开展现场抽查,在全国范围内开展"儿童青少年预防近视"系列主题宣传活动。

在"视觉 2020"行动倡议的推动下,我国的防盲治盲工作取得了重大进展。我国各级政府重视防盲工作,在防盲工作中发挥了主导作用[17]。我国县级医院眼科防治服务体系逐步完善,县级眼科机构数量持续增多、质量不断加强;眼科医务人员队伍不断壮大,人力资源数量质量不断优化;白内障、沙眼等主要致盲性眼病的防治成效显著;眼科设备配置日趋完善,我国眼健康事业取得了飞速的进展。

参 考 文 献

1. World Health Organization. What is VISION 2020? [EB/OL].[2020-04-19]. https://www. who. int/blindness/ partnerships/vision2020/en/.

2. The International Agency for the Prevention of Blindness. VISION 2020 Action Plan 2006-2011.[EB/OL]. [2020-04-19]. https://www. iapb. org/resources/vision-2020-action-plan-2006-2011/.

3. The International Agency for the Prevention of Blindness. What is VISION 2020? [EB/OL].[2020-04-19], https://www. iapb. org/global-initiatives/vision-2020/what-is-vision-2020/.

4. 何守志. 21 世纪白内障复明工作面临挑战 [J]. 中华眼科杂志, 2001, 37 (5): 321-324.

5. 中国防盲治盲网. "视觉 2020" 简介 [EB/OL].(2013-01-01)[2020-04-17]. http://moheyes. com/News/Details/ a8e735ab-32a9-4a38-a060-b269b9f24215.

6. 赵家良. 促进普遍的眼健康,推动我国防盲工作持续发展 [J]. 中华眼科杂志, 2014, 50 (3): 161-163.

7. 胡翔, 张睿, 徐笑, 等. 凝心聚力开创我国防盲治盲工作新局面 [J]. 中华医学杂志, 2013, 93 (47): 3731-3732.

8. 中华人民共和国国家卫生健康委员会. 国家卫生计生委关于印发"十三五"全国眼健康规划 (2016-2020 年) 的 通 知 (国 卫 医 发〔2016〕57 号)[EB/OL].(2016-11-09)[2020-04-19]. http://www. nhc. gov. cn/wjw/

ghjh/201611/9463afb00ac84910bb3c22f8629cf90a. shtml.

9. 杨晓慧, 胡爱莲, 王宁利. 从防盲治盲到全面的眼健康 [J]. 眼科, 2017 (1): 9-11.

10. 王宇. 中国眼科现状调查统计分析报告 (2003) 发行 [Z]. 2004.

11. World Health Organization. 普遍的眼健康: 2014-2019 年全球行动计划.[EB/OL].(2013-05-24)[2020-04-19]. https://apps. who. int/iris/bitstream/handle/10665/105937/9789245506560_chi. pdf; jsessionid=938CF4336F6ED37306821D82CE8076BB? sequence=9.

12. 管怀进. 我国防盲与眼科流行病学研究的现状及发展 [J]. 中华眼科杂志, 2010, 46 (10): 938-943.

13. 王宁利, 胡爱莲. 我国沙眼防治的启迪与思考 [J]. 中华眼科杂志, 2015 (7): 484-486.

14. Gogate P, Muhit M, 石磊. 发展中国家的儿童盲与白内障 [J]. 实用防盲技术, 2010, 5 (3): 93-95.

15. Chen Y, Feng J, Li F, et al. Analysis of changes in characteristics of severe retinopathy of prematurity patients after screening guidelines were issued in China [J]. Retina, 2015, 35 (8): 1674-1679.

16. 中华人民共和国国家卫生健康委员会. 卫生部关于印发《早产儿治疗用氧和视网膜病变防治指南》的通知 (卫医发〔2004〕104 号)[EB/OL].(2004-06-28)[2020-04-19]. http://www. nhc. gov. cn/bgt/pw10405/200406/21c22c38dc004863bb5af817fb7753d0. shtml.

17. 赵家良. 中国眼科医师要坚定不移地推进 "视觉 2020" 行动 [J]. 实用医院临床杂志, 2011, 7 (6): 1-3.

眼科资源是人人享有眼健康的关键,提高眼科资源可及性是落实防盲治盲工作的重要环节。20 年来,我国眼健康事业飞速发展,眼科资源的建设取得了显著进展,县级医院眼科防治服务体系增强、眼科人力资源数量质量不断优化、眼科设备配置逐渐完善。

一、县级眼科机构数量增多、服务能力加强

提升县级医院综合能力是提高我国医疗服务整体能力、引领县级医院发展的重要举措。着力县级医疗机构眼科专科建设是我国实现“视觉 2020”总目标的关键。在我国各项防盲政策与项目的不断推动下,县级医疗机构充分利用眼健康相关支持项目,通过鼓励并支持基层人员参加眼科专业培训、进修学习,开展各类眼病筛查工作,显著提高了自身的眼健康服务能力。2003 年,我国可提供眼科医疗服务的县级医院和设有独立眼科的县级医院分别为 1 995 所和 1 033 所[1]。2014 年,我国可提供眼科医疗服务的县级医院以及设有独立眼科的县级医院分别为 3 359 所和 1 463 所[2,3]。在各项防盲政策的推动下,我国县级医院的眼科医疗机构蓬勃发展,据 2018 年全国眼科资源调查显示:我国目前可提供眼科医疗服务的县级医院以及设有独立眼科的县级医院分别为 3 478 所和 1 807 所(图 4-1)。超过 10% 的县级医院在 2014—2018 年间设立单独眼科。基层眼科医疗团队更加专业,医疗服务更加优质,为我国基层眼科防盲事业提供了更多实践平台。随着眼科医疗机构数量的增多、质量的增强,县级医院总门诊服务人次也逐年攀升,从 2003 年的 941 万人次到 2014 年的 3 140 万人次[1,2],2018 年县级医院眼科门诊量达到 6 419 万人次,约为 2014 年的 2 倍。越来越多的患者享受到了便利的基层眼科服务。

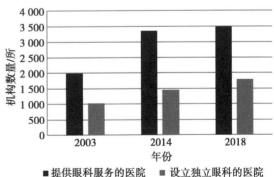

图 4-1　我国县级医院 2003、2014 及 2018 年眼科机构情况

二、眼科人员队伍不断壮大完善

从"十五"到"十三五",在防盲政策的支持与防盲项目的推动下,我国眼科专业队伍日益壮大,为推动防盲治盲工作开展和为人民群众提供眼保健服务提供了坚实的人力资源保障。据调查显示:我国眼科医师的数量由2003年的1.91万人发展到2006年的2.83万人,再至2014年的3.63万人[1,3](图4-2),2018年全国眼科医疗机构统计结果显示,这一数据已达到4.48万人。此外县级医院眼科医师规模也得到了很大的提升。县级医院眼科医师的数量由1998年的8 769人发展至2003年的9 965人到2014年的1.32万人[1,3,4](图4-3),直至2018年的1.42万人。中、高级医师占比由1998年的45.35%提升至2014年的59.73%,眼科医生职称结构愈加合理[3,4]。我国政府一直大力推进白内障防盲工作,自20世纪80年代起,就在各项防盲规划与防盲政策中明确不同阶段我国白内障防盲的努力目标和措施。大力加强县级综合医院眼科能力建设,县级医院白内障手术能力得到了很大的提升。2018年我国具备白内障手术能力的医生是13 835人,是2000年(5 939人)的2.33倍[5](图4-4)。目前,我国眼科医师总数已经达到4.48万人,即每5万人中有1.6名眼科医生[6],已超过WHO对亚洲地区每5万人中应有1个眼科医生的要求[7]。

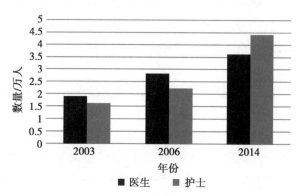

图 4-2 我国 2003、2006 及 2014 年眼科医师、护士数量

护理工作者是眼科卫生服务的重要主体之一,其数量和结构不但决定着眼科护理工作质量,又直接关系到医疗质量和医疗安全。自1999年我国参与WHO"视觉2020"行动倡议后,在各项政策推动下,我国眼科专职护士数量大幅提升。2003年我国眼科护士为1.61万人,2006年为2.24万人,至2014年已达到4.41万人[1,8],(图4-2)。尤其县级医院从事眼科护理的人员也从1998年的7 886人,发展至2003年的7 978人,到2014年的1.54万人[1,2,4],(图4-3)。同时,眼科医护比逐渐趋于合理,2014年眼科医护比为1:1.21,比起2006年的1:0.79,8年间提高了53.16%[2]。

未矫正的屈光不正是全球视觉损伤的主要原因之一,占比约42%[9]。2018年全国儿童青少年总体近视率为53.6%。其中,6岁儿童为14.5%,小学生为36.0%,初中生为71.6%,高中生为81.0%[10]。我国学生近视呈现高发、低龄化趋势。在国家各项防盲政策的推动下,我国视光师的数量从2006年的1 487人增长到了2014年的3 950名,增长了1.5倍[3](图4-5)。2014—2018年共增加了2 468人,即从2014年的3 950人上升到2018年的6 418人,增长了近1倍。但相对于我国庞大的近视患病群体来说,合格的专职验光师仍然存在较大缺口,培养专业验光师的工作依然任重道远。

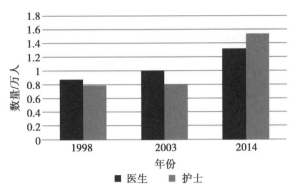

图 4-3　我国县级医院 1998、2003 及
2014 年眼科医生、护士数量

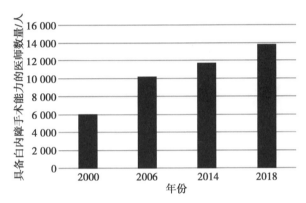

图 4-4　2000、2006、2014、2018 年具备
白内障手术能力的医师数量

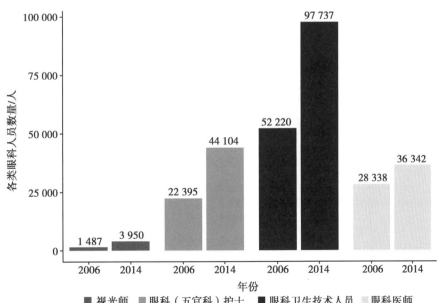

图 4-5　我国 2006 年、2014 年眼科医生、护士、视光师数量

三、眼科设备配置逐渐完善

2016 年,国家发布《县医院医疗服务能力基本标准》和《县医院医疗服务能力推荐标准》(国卫办医发〔2016〕12 号),这两项标准对县医院包括眼科等临床科室的医疗技术水平、设备设施作出了明确的规定。眼科设备作为眼科资源的重要组成部分,是提升基层眼保健服务的关键。随着我国县级医院眼科医疗机构,眼科专业人员的不断增加,各医院眼科设备的配置也愈加完善。非接触眼压计、眼科 A/B 超、超声乳化仪、手术显微镜等眼科设备配置率显著增长。2015 年,超过 80% 的县级医院配备非接触眼压计、手术显微镜、直接检眼镜、间接检眼镜。接近一半的县级医院配备超声乳化仪与视野仪[1,11](表 4-1、图 4-6)。

表 4-1　我国眼科设备配置率 2003 年与 2015 年情况对比　　　　　　　　　单位:%

年份	眼压计	间接检眼镜	直接检眼镜	眼科A/B超	超声乳化仪	手术显微镜	视野仪
2003 年	80.9	39.8	63.5	25.7	12.1	61.0	33.1
2015 年	89.6	42.9	84.2	76.0	44.4	83.4	40.7

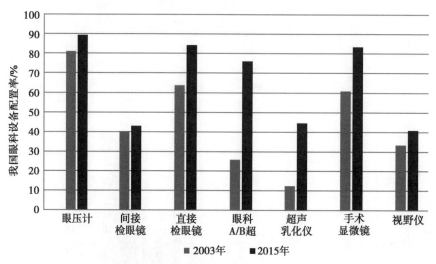

图 4-6　我国眼科设备配置率 2003 年与 2015 年情况对比

参 考 文 献

1. 王宇. 中国眼科现状调查统计分析报告 (2003) 发行 [Z]. 2004.
2. 冯晶晶, 安磊, 王志锋, 等. 2014 年我国大陆地区县级医疗机构眼科人力资源配置和服务提供现况调查 [J]. 中华眼科杂志, 2018, 54 (12): 929-934.
3. Zhan L., Safaya N., Erkou H., et al. A comparative analysis on human resources among the specialized

ophthalmic medical institutions in China [J]. Human Resources for Health, 2020, 18 (1): 29.

4. 张文斌, 刘建军. 我国县级医院眼科卫生资源及卫生服务利用效益评价 [J]. 医学与社会, 2001, 14 (6): 57-59.

5. 徐海峰, 张文斌. 2000 年我国眼科资源现状调查研究 [J]. 医学与社会, 2005, 18 (5): 7-9.

6. 中华人民共和国国家统计局. 中华人民共和国 2017 年国民经济和社会发展统计公报.[EB/OL].(2018-02-28)[2020-04-15]. http://www. stats. gov. cn/tjsj/zxfb/201802/t20180228_1585631. html.

7. Thylefors B. A global initiative for the elimination of avoidable blindness [J]. Community Eye Health, 1998, 11 (25): 1-3.

8. 景正伟, 任贺, 王洪源, 等. 中国眼科护理人力资源配置分析 [J]. 中华现代护理杂志, 2019, 25 (6): 703-707.

9. World Health Organization. 普遍的眼健康: 2014-2019 年全球行动计划.[EB/OL].(2013-05-24)[2020-04-19]. https://apps. who. int/iris/bitstream/handle/10665/105937/9789245506560_chi. pdf; jsessionid=938CF4336F6ED37306821D82CE8076BB？sequence=9.

10. 中华人民共和国国家卫生健康委员会宣传司. 儿童青少年总体近视率为 53.6% 我国将更有针对性地开展近视干预 [EB/OL].(2019-05-08)[2020-04-15]. http://www. nhc. gov. cn/xcs/s7847/201905/11c679a40eb3494cade977f65f1c3740. shtml

11. 廖鹏, 徐笑, 景正伟, 等. 全国县医院眼科设备配置分析 [J]. 中国医院管理 2019, 39 (4): 62-65.

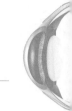

第五章 盲和视力损伤大幅度下降

2016年全国卫生与健康大会强调,要把人民健康放在优先发展的战略地位上。眼健康是身心健康的重要组成部分,然而现阶段盲和视力损伤依然严重影响我国居民的眼健康。据2006年第二次全国残疾人抽样调查显示:中国有视力残疾人1 233万[1],占全国残疾人总数的14.86%。

多年来,在国家卫生健康委的领导下,在全国防盲技术指导组的技术支持下,以及全国各级防盲工作人员的不断努力下,我国从各个层面不断深入开展防盲治盲工作。一是充分利用全国爱眼日、世界视觉日、世界青光眼周等健康宣传日开展宣传活动,努力提高民众的自我防控意识;组织编写和出版适用于基层防盲工作的书籍和对群众进行防盲教育的宣传品;积极利用报刊、广播、电视、网络等形式开展多样化的防盲治盲的宣教工作,促进全社会重视眼健康工作;二是大力弘扬"大医精诚、救死扶伤"的优良传统,深入报道广大眼科医务人员和基层医疗卫生工作者深入贫困地区为贫困群众解除眼病、重见光明的生动事迹,在全社会营造了积极参与防盲治盲工作的良好舆论氛围;三是重视白内障患者复明工作,尤其是贫困人口的白内障复明工作。依托各类防盲治盲项目,为基层、偏远地区数百万患者输送了光明;四是依托"中国县级医院眼科团队培训项目"等,在不断完善我国防盲治盲工作体系的基础上,构建适合我国国情、较为完善的眼科医疗服务网络,从而为国民提供全面、公平、可及的眼科医疗服务;五是通过全国、各省(自治区、直辖市)、市防盲技术指导组网络,不断加强和促进各地区之间的合作与交流,不断总结防盲治盲经验,例如,通过眼健康简讯、出版刊物和定期召开区域性或全国性会议交流防盲工作经验;六是通过定期开展各种形式的全国性讲习班或培训班,培训省(自治区、直辖市)、市及地区的防盲骨干。

这些工作改善了我国盲和视力损伤的现状:2006年和2014年我国卫生部门组织开展了两次九省(自治区、直辖市)盲和视力损伤流行病学调查,结果显示:按照最佳矫正视力进行评估,我国50岁以上人群中,中重度视力损伤的患病率从2006年的10.8%下降到2014年的10.3%,下降幅度达4.6%;此外,盲率从2006年的2.29%下降至2014年的1.66%,下降幅度达27.5%[2]。结合2010年全国人口普查数据,我们很容易估算:仅在50岁以上人群中,我国就减少了数百万盲人。这些数据表明,我国盲和视力损伤的患病率均实现了大幅度下降,我国的防盲治盲工作已经取得了重大进展。

—————— 参 考 文 献 ——————

1. 中华人民共和国国家统计局. 2006 年第二次全国残疾人抽样调查主要数据公报.[EB/OL].(2006-12-01) [2020-06-17]. http://www. gov. cn/ztzl/gacjr/content_459223. htm

2. Zhao J, Xu X, Ellwein L B, et al. Causes of Visual Impairment and Blindness in the 2006 and 2014 Nine-Province Surveys in Rural China [J]. AM J OPHTHALMOL, 2019 (197): 80-87.

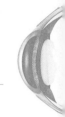

第六章　主要致盲性眼病疾病谱变化

　　随着我国防盲工作的推进、国家经济水平的提升、人民生活方式的改变以及我国人口结构的改变,致盲性眼病疾病谱随之发生了重大改变,主要致盲性眼病已由过去的沙眼传染性眼病转变为以白内障、角膜病、视网膜疾病、屈光不正、青光眼以及弱视为主的代谢性和年龄相关性非传染性眼病。

一、白内障

　　"十三五"期间,每百万人口白内障手术例数(Cataract surgical rate,CSR)、白内障手术脱残率均有所提高,但随着我国步入老龄化社会,老年人眼健康需求将显著增加。40岁以上人群是白内障等年龄相关性眼病的高危群体。在60~69岁老年人群中患病率接近50%,而70岁以上老年人群中,患病率则高达79.2%[1]。2017年,我国60岁及以上老年人口有2.41亿人,占总人口的17.3%[2],预计到2050年将达到4.8亿人,作为高患病率、高伤残率、高医疗利用率的老年患者群体,眼健康问题将显著增加,白内障目前仍是我国首位致盲性眼病,因此,我国防盲治盲的主要工作任务是继续提高CSR,增加手术覆盖率、提高手术质量。

二、角膜相关疾病

　　在我国,角膜相关疾病是仅次于白内障的第二大致盲性眼病,且角膜相关疾病的致盲风险较其他眼病更高,角膜相关疾病患者的致盲率超过70%[3]。角膜相关疾病的诊治和角膜盲的防控是我国眼健康工作的重要内容,尤其是感染性角膜病。

　　近年来,我国不断拓宽角膜供体来源:除传统的角膜捐献方式外,还拓展了采用激光近视手术中余留的角膜板层材料、发展人工角膜材料等。现在,每年通过角膜移植手术复明的患者已接近1万例[4],较20世纪90年代的1 000例有了大幅上涨。不过考虑到患者的基数,1万例尚远远不能满足需求,未来角膜盲的工作重点依然是增加角膜供体来源和培养角膜病专科医师。

三、黄斑病变、糖尿病视网膜病变等视网膜疾病

随着人们的生活水平不断提高、生活方式的改变,慢性病的发病率也逐年增高,因而与之相关的眼底疾病,如高血压眼底病变、糖尿病视网膜病变、年龄相关性黄斑变性等的患病人数大幅增加。由于病因复杂、病期长等原因,眼底病已逐渐成为重要的不可逆性致盲原因。

早期筛查和早期控制是眼底疾病的有效干预措施:糖尿病视网膜病变被称为首位可预防的致盲眼底病变,通过早期筛查、定期随访和适时的激光治疗可以有效地避免致盲以及视力损害,抗血管内皮生长因子(anti-vascular endothelial growth factor,anti-VEGF)治疗的广泛应用可以使患者延缓病情发展,恢复部分视功能。目前我国已经将雷珠单抗、阿柏西普、康柏西普等 anti-VEGF 药物纳入医保目录。数据显示:我国每 10 个 20 周岁以上成人中就有 1 名糖尿病患者[5]。糖尿病的高患病率意味着糖尿病视网膜病变的高患病率及大量的糖尿病视网膜病变致盲患者。据统计,我国糖尿病视网膜病变在总人群的发病率为 1.3%[6]。在未来一段时间内,眼底病的筛查将成为今后眼健康工作的重点,目前已有很多机构在开展此类工作,例如由全国防盲技术指导组与中国微循环学会主办的旨在"提高糖网病筛查率,避免糖尿病患者失明"的"中国糖网筛防工程",截至 2019 年 11 月,中国糖网筛防工程覆盖医院近 577 家(其中三甲医院 200 多家),遍及 29 个省(自治区、直辖市),共筛查 80 万余名糖尿病患者。

四、屈光不正

近视是屈光不正的主要类型,其中高度近视所致的并发症可导致视力低下甚至致盲。在我国某些地区,高度近视相关的视网膜病变已经成为成人不可逆性致盲性眼病的首要原因,因此近视防控已成为我国眼健康工作的重要内容。调查显示,全国儿童青少年总体近视率为 53.6%[7],而某些地区的大学生近视的患病率已超 90%[8],高度近视的患病率达 10% 以上[8,9]。此外,未矫正的中高度远视及散光也可影响儿童正常的视觉发育,可能导致斜视及弱视的发生,也会影响正常视功能的建立。

解决屈光不正引起的视力问题最简便的方法是配戴合适的眼镜,我国通过增加验光配镜的人力资源、提供质优价廉的眼镜和方便可及的验光服务等措施,正努力改善屈光不正导致的盲和视力损伤问题。

五、青光眼

我国人群中,青光眼的患病率高达 2.58%,到 2020 年预计患者数将达到 2 516 万[10]。青光眼的发病凶险,发病机理不清,缺乏病因学治疗。临床上青光眼患者的病因大多隐匿复杂,容易延误治疗。尤其是原发性开角型青光眼,其发病隐匿,早期诊断困难,检出率低,多

数患者初次就诊时已经伴有明显的视神经损伤,致使致盲率一直居高不下。近年来随着我国各地区不断推广适宜技术,青光眼的致盲率已经较 20 世纪 90 年代有了大幅下降,其中急性闭角型青光眼的致盲率已经从 20 世纪 90 年代的 50%[11] 下降到了近年来的 14.5%。开角型青光眼的检出率则从 10% 上升到 40%。

但是鉴于青光眼所导致的盲具有不可逆性,且大众对青光眼的防范意识不足,临床亟需加强相关科普宣传教育,对青光眼做到早发现、早治疗。此外,基层医院的医师培训也应将其作为工作重点:基层医院大部分缺乏专科青光眼医师,手术治疗仍以小梁切除术为主,术后远期效果较差,部分患者缺乏规范化随访,最终仍不能避免失明。因此,在强调早发现、加大普查力度的同时,还需强调规范化随访,尤其是针对原发性开角型青光眼以及慢性闭角型青光眼。未来应加强对基层眼科医师进行青光眼专科知识的培训,除眼压外,还需重视眼底照相、视野检查、光学相干断层扫描仪等在青光眼患者规范化随访管理中的应用。自 2017 年开始,世界青光眼周连续三年强调眼底检查的重要性,未来借助人工智能等手段开展以社区为基础的青光眼高危人群筛查,将会成为青光眼防治工作的重点。

六、弱视

我国 3~6 岁儿童弱视患病率约为 2.8%,6~14 岁少年儿童患病率约为 3.5%。儿童时期是视觉发育的关键期和敏感期,开展儿童时期斜视、屈光不正、屈光参差等弱视相关危险因素的筛查是弱视早发现、早治疗的关键。2013 年,为了早发现影响儿童视觉发育眼病,尽早矫治、及时转诊,预防儿童可控制性眼病的发生发展,保护和促进儿童视功能正常发育,国家卫生行政部门印发了《儿童眼及视力保健技术规范》。该规范明确规定了儿童应定期接受眼病筛查和视力评估,并注意用眼卫生,防止眼外伤和预防传染性眼病[12-14]。

通过国家卫生行业专项项目"常见致盲性眼病的筛查、诊断和干预技术的标准化与应用研究"、国际奥比斯组织国际重大合作项目"津滇两地少年儿童斜视、弱视及屈光不正的流行病学研究"等以人群为基础的大样本儿童斜视弱视与视力发育的流行病学调查研究的实施,以及我国斜视与小儿眼科专家经多次会议充分讨论后《弱视诊断专家共识》的形成,学龄前儿童弱视诊断扩大化的情况以及因过度诊断导致的过度治疗所造成不必要的医疗资源的浪费在逐渐减少。尽管如此,由于弱视的患病率高达约 3%[15],弱视的早发现、早干预仍然是儿童盲与低视力防治中的关键内容。

参 考 文 献

1. 袁贤斌, 张栋彦, 陈盛举, 等. 甘肃省不同海拔地区 50 岁以上人群白内障患病率调查 [J]. 中华眼科杂志, 2019, 55 (8): 589-594.
2. 中国防盲治盲网. 2017 年中国白内障复明手术报送情况排名 [EB/OL].(2018-03-28)[2020-05-13]. http://www. moheyes. com/News/Details/3bed4465-7e8c-40e3-8532-25eeb128565b.

3. 高华, 陈秀念, 史伟云. 我国盲的患病率及主要致盲性疾病状况分析 [J]. 中华眼科杂志, 2019, 55 (8): 625-628.

4. 史伟云, 谢立信. 我国角膜病领域的学术发展方向 [J]. 中华眼科杂志, 2014, 50 (9): 641-645.

5. Yang W, Lu J, Weng J, et al. Prevalence of diabetes among men and women in China [J]. N Engl J Med, 2010, 362 (12): 1090-1101.

6. 中华医学会眼科学会眼底病学组. 我国糖尿病视网膜病变临床诊疗指南 (2014 年)[J]. 中华眼科杂志, 2014, 50 (11): 851-865.

7. 中华人民共和国国家卫生健康委员会宣传司. 儿童青少年总体近视率为 53.6% 我国将更有针对性地开展近视干预 [EB/OL].(2019-05-08)[2020-04-15]. http://www. nhc. gov. cn/xcs/s7847/201905/11c679a40eb3494cade977f65f1c3740. shtml.

8. Dong L, Kang Y, Li Y, et al. Prevalence and time trends of myopia in children and adolescents in China: A Systemic Review and Meta-Analysis [J]. Retina, 2020, 40 (3): 399-411.

9. Sun J, Zhou J, Zhao P, et al. High prevalence of myopia and high myopia in 5060 Chinese university students in Shanghai [J]. Invest Ophthalmol Vis Sci, 2012 (53): 7504-7509.

10. Song P, Wang J, Bucan K, et al. National and subnational prevalence and burden of glaucoma in China: A systematic analysis [J]. J Glob Health, 2017, 7 (2): 20705.

11. 李惠民. 湘潭县农村原发性青光眼致盲率调查 [J]. 湖南医学, 1986 (3): 158.

12. 赵堪兴. 早期发现和早期干预, 努力提高弱视的防治水平 [J]. 中华眼科杂志, 2002, 38 (8): 449-451.

13. 赵堪兴, 郑曰忠. 我国弱视临床防治中亟待的问题 [J]. 中华眼科杂志, 2009, 45 (11): 961-962.

14. 赵堪兴, 史学锋. 重视婴幼儿视力异常的筛查 [J]. 中华眼科杂志, 2013, 49 (7): 577-579.

15. 中华人民共和国国家卫生健康委员会医政医管局. 弱视是可避免的严重的视觉损伤性疾病, 我国弱视患者约有 4000 万 [EB/OL].(2018-06-05)[2020-05-19]. http://www. nhc. gov. cn/yzygj/s7652/201806/f8477829bfe149aebe4d75ddce0a663e. shtml.

第七章　近视防控

一、我国儿童青少年近视的现状

屈光不正已成为全球视力损伤的主要原因,是 WHO 在全球消除可避免盲和视力损害的 5 种眼病之一[1,2],而近视性屈光不正是引起未矫正的视力损伤的主要原因[3]。据统计,全球近视者到 2050 年将高达 47.58 亿,占全球总人口的 49.8%[4]。近年来,随着经济社会发展和知识性竞争加剧,我国儿童青少年的近视患病率居高不下,而且呈现出"发病年龄提前、患病率急剧上升、近视进展快和程度高"等特点,已成为危害我国儿童青少年眼健康的重要公共卫生问题。

根据全国各地的调查,近视的患病率随年龄和地区呈现较大差异。上海对学龄前儿童开展的调查发现 4 岁、5 岁、6 岁儿童的近视患病率已达 2.3%、3.5% 和 5.2%[5]。在中小学生中,近视的患病率陡然升高。广州地区调查发现,一到九年级学生近视的平均患病率为 47.4%,汉族为 48.9%,其他民族为 35.6%[6],近视患病率从一年级的 0.2% 增长至九年级的 68.4%。在河南安阳地区开展的调查中,一年级和七年级近视患病率依次为 3.9% 和 67.3%[7],而此地大学生人群中近视的患病率达 83.2%,其中高度近视高达 11.1%[8]。

此外,根据邯郸眼病研究调查结果,此地区 30 岁以上成年人的近视患病率仅为 26.7%,高度近视患病率仅为 1.8%[9]。综合对比成年人的近视率,这代儿童青少年近视的患病率已经远超过去。

2018 年下半年,国家卫生健康委会同教育部、民政部组织开展了 2018 年全国儿童青少年近视调查工作。本次调查共覆盖了全国 1 033 所幼儿园、3 810 所中小学校,共筛查 111.74 万人。2019 年 4 月 29 日,国家卫生健康委举办新闻发布会,介绍 2018 年儿童青少年近视调查结果。调查结果显示,2018 年全国儿童青少年总体近视率为 53.6%[10]。其中 6 岁儿童为 14.5%,小学生为 36.0%,初中生为 71.6%,高中生为 81.0%。此外,低年龄段近视问题比较突出,在小学和初中阶段,近视率随着年级的升高快速增长。小学阶段从一年级的 15.7% 增长到六年级的 59.0%。初中阶段从初一年级的 64.9% 增长到初三年级的 77.0%,高三年级高度近视(近视度数超过 600 度)的人数,在近视总数中占比达到 21.9%。

二、近视防控的国家战略

近视不仅会给日常生活和学习带来诸多不便,近视尤其是高度近视,还可能导致青光眼、白内障、视网膜脱离和黄斑变性等严重并发症,危害视觉健康甚至导致失明[11]。因此,近视防控问题是我国政府关注的重要问题。

近年来,党中央、国务院高度重视儿童青少年近视防控工作,近视防控已成为国家战略。2016 年至 2019 年,连续 4 年将全国"爱眼日"的主题聚焦在儿童青少年的近视防控,分别是"呵护眼睛,从小做起""'目'浴阳光,预防近视""科学防控近视、关爱孩子眼健康"和"共同呵护好孩子的眼睛,让他们拥有一个光明的未来"。为做好近视的防治工作,2018 年 6 月 5 日,国家卫生健康委召开专题新闻发布会,介绍儿童青少年科学防控近视情况,同时发布了《近视防治指南》《弱视诊治指南》和《斜视诊治指南》三部指南,一方面是为了指导医疗机构和眼科医务人员提高服务能力;另一方面意在引导学生和家长树立正确用眼的意识。为明确各地儿童青少年近视率基数,国家卫生健康委办公厅、教育部办公厅、财政部办公厅联合发布了《关于开展 2018 年儿童青少年近视调查工作的通知》(国卫办疾控函〔2018〕932 号)。

2018 年 8 月 28 日,习近平总书记作出重要指示,强调全社会都要行动起来,共同呵护好孩子的眼睛,让他们拥有一个光明的未来。为贯彻落实这一重要指示精神,切实加强新时代儿童青少年近视防控工作,2018 年 8 月 30 日,教育部、国家卫生健康委、体育总局、财政部、人力资源和社会保障部、市场监管总局、国家新闻出版署、广电总局八部门制定了《综合防控儿童青少年近视实施方案》[12](教体艺〔2018〕3 号)(以下简称《实施方案》)。《实施方案》不仅明确了家庭、学校、医疗卫生机构、学生、政府相关部门应采取的防控措施,还明确了八个部门防控近视的职责和任务。《实施方案》强调,各省级人民政府主要负责同志要亲自抓近视防控工作。建立全国儿童青少年近视防控工作评议考核制度,核实各地 2018 年儿童青少年近视率,2019 年起对各省级人民政府进行评议考核,结果向社会公布。

2019 年,国家卫生健康委联合教育部门在全国开展"儿童青少年预防近视"系列主题宣传活动,提升了儿童青少年健康素养水平。国家卫生健康委疾控局组织制定并印发了《儿童青少年近视防控适宜技术指南》,指导科学规范开展防控工作,提高防控技术能力。教育部办公厅印发了《关于公布 2018 年全国儿童青少年近视防控试点县(市、区)和改革试验区遴选结果名单的通知》(教体艺厅函〔2018〕77 号),命名北京市东城区等 84 个地区为全国儿童青少年近视防控试点县(市、区),天津市北辰区等 29 个地区为全国儿童青少年近视防控改革试验区。全国防盲技术指导组组织编写的《儿童青少年近视防治科普 100 问》,对近视防治中的疑问和误区给出了科学解释。此外,为了做到科学防控、精准施策,针对不同年龄组的儿童青少年,国家卫生健康委疾控局和首都医科大学附属北京同仁医院(以下简称"北京同仁医院")联合编写了《幼儿园防控近视手册》《小学生防控近视手册》《初中生防控近视手册》《高中生防控近视手册》。目前,在全社会已营造了儿童青少年近视防控"政府主导、部门配合、专家指导、学校教育、家庭关注"的良好氛围。

三、综合防控措施

针对儿童青少年近视的特点,我国已采取多种措施对近视开展综合防控。如严格落实国家基本公共卫生服务中关于 0~6 岁儿童眼保健和视力检查工作要求,建立屈光发育档案,做到早监测、早发现、早预警、早干预。规范诊断治疗,县级及以上综合医院普遍开展眼科医疗服务,认真落实《近视防治指南》等诊疗规范,不断提高眼健康服务能力。加强健康教育,从健康教育入手,加强中小学生近视筛查及普查,发动儿童青少年和家长自主健康行动。积极开展近视防治相关研究,加强防治近视科研成果与技术的应用与全面推广。

针对众多环境因素对近视发生和发展的影响,如户外活动缺乏、电子产品的过度使用、用眼习惯不良等,采取了增加户外活动和锻炼,积极引导儿童青少年进行户外活动或体育锻炼,控制儿童青少年电子产品的使用等干预措施,避免不良用眼行为,保持"一尺、一拳、一寸"[13]。严格依据国家课程方案和课程标准组织安排教学活动,不要盲目参加课外培训,根据孩子兴趣爱好合理选择。坚持眼保健操等护眼措施,保障睡眠和营养。针对已近视儿童,开展科学的诊疗与矫正,如配戴框架眼镜或角膜塑形镜、使用低浓度阿托品等[14]。

<hr />

参 考 文 献

1. Pascolini D, Mariotti S. Global estimates of visual impairment: 2010 [J]. Br J Ophthalmol, 2012, 96 (5): 614-618.

2. Zhao J, Xu X, Ellwein L, et al. Prevalence of Vision Impairment in Older Adults in Rural China in 2014 and Comparisons With the 2006 China Nine-Province Survey [J]. Am J Ophthalmol, 2018, 185 (1): 81-93.

3. Xu L, Wang Y, Li Y, et al. Causes of blindness and visual impairment in urban and rural areas in Beijing: the Beijing Eye Study [J]. Ophthalmology, 2006, 113 (7): 1134-1137.

4. Holden B, Fricke T, Wilson D, et al. Global Prevalence of Myopia and High Myopiaand Temporal Trends from 2000 through 2050 [J]. Ophthalmology, 2016, 123 (5): 1036-1042.

5. Ma Y, Qu X, Zhu X, et al. Age-Specific Prevalence of Visual Impairment and Refractive Error in Children Aged 3-10 Years in Shanghai, China [J]. Invest Ophthalmol Vis Sci, 2016, 57 (14): 6188-6196.

6. Guo L, Yang J, Mai J, et al. Prevalence and associated factors of myopia among primary and middle school-aged students: a school-based study in Guangzhou [J]. Eye, 2016, 30 (6): 796-804.

7. Li S, Liu L, Li S, et al. Design, methodology and baseline data of a school-based cohort study in Central China: the Anyang Childhood Eye Study [J]. Ophthalmic Epidemiol, 2013, 20 (6): 348-359.

8. Wei S, Sun Y, Li S, et al. Refractive Errors in University Students in Central China: The Anyang University Students Eye Study [J]. Invest Ophthalmol Vis Sci, 2018, 59 (11): 4691-4700.

9. Liang Y, Wong T, Sun L, et al. Refractive errors in a rural Chinese adult population the Handan eye study [J]. Ophthalmology, 2009, 116 (11): 2119-2127.

10. 中华人民共和国国家卫生健康委员会宣传司. 儿童青少年总体近视率为 53.6% 我国将更有针对性地开展近视干预 [EB/OL].(2019-05-08)[2020-04-15]. http://www. nhc. gov. cn/xcs/s7847/201905/11c679a40eb3494cade977f65f1c3740. shtml.

11. Saw S, Gazzard G, Shih-Yen E, et al. Myopia and associated pathological complications [J]. Ophthalmic Physiol Opt, 2005, 25 (5): 381-391.

12. 中华人民共和国教育部, 中华人民共和国国家卫生健康委员会, 中华人民共和国国家体育总局, 等. 教育部等八部门关于印发《综合防控儿童青少年近视实施方案》(教体艺〔2018〕3 号) 的通知. [EB/OL].(2018-08-30)[2020-04-05]. http://www. moe. gov. cn/srcsite/A17/moe_943/s3285/201808/ t20180830_346672. html.

13. Li S, Li S, Kang M, et al. Near Work Related Parameters and Myopia in Chinese Children: the Anyang Childhood Eye Study [J]. PLoS One, 2015, 10 (8): e0134514.

14. Walline J, Lindsley K, Vedula S, et al. Interventions to slow progression of myopia in children [J]. Cochrane Database Syst Rev, 2020 (1): CD004916.

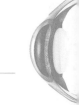

第八章 消灭致盲性沙眼

一、中华人民共和国成立初期,"十人九沙"

中华人民共和国成立前后,沙眼在我国广泛流行,是我国首位致盲病因。"十人九沙"是当时沙眼在我国广泛流行的真实写照。综合全国各地的统计数字,从不同职业来看,工人患沙眼者约为 40%~70%,农民约为 40%~80%,学生约为 30%~70%。从不同地域来说,在长江以南和沿海一带,约为 30%~50%,长江以北、长城以南等地区约为 40%~70%,东北地区约为 50%~80%,兰州等地沙眼发病率高于我国其他地区,约为 60%~90%。沙眼使视力减退者约占 55.8%,致盲者 7%,共计 62.8%[1]。

二、群防群治,科研助力,成效显著

中华人民共和国成立初期,沙眼作为最主要致盲性眼病,被纳入国家公共卫生规划之中。1956 年,防治沙眼纳入《1956 年到 1967 年全国农业发展纲要》并于 1957 年 10 月正式公布修正草案。1957—1959 年,国家进一步开展防治沙眼与改厕运动,切断沙眼传播途径[1]。1958 年国家发布《全国沙眼防治规划》[2],指出防治沙眼工作的方针任务为坚持依靠群众,结合爱国卫生运动,推行讲卫生为中心的综合防治措施。规划明确提出了沙眼防治的具体措施:提倡一人一巾,经常保持毛巾的清洁;推广流水洗脸、改变一家人合用一个脸盆甚至是一盆水的情况;注意保护眼睛,不要用手揉眼睛,勤洗手脸;注意改善水质,保持用水清洁;对服务性行业进行严格的卫生监督,加强管理;提高工厂、学校、托儿所等集体生活单位的集体预防意识,防治沙眼的传播。同时,规划指出防治沙眼必须防与治紧密结合,防和治是解决沙眼问题最重要的两个方面,要坚持综合性的措施。加强防沙眼宣传教育与卫生教育,开展经常性宣传教育工作,把防治沙眼的办法教给群众。

由于病原体不明,沙眼曾被称为不明病因的"眼科黑暗区域"[3]。为了更有效地开展沙眼防治工作,眼科科学工作者积极响应政府号召,投身沙眼防治工作。1955 年 8 月,汤飞凡教授和张晓楼教授在世界上首次成功分离出沙眼病原体——"沙眼衣原体",开启了全世界沙眼研究和防治沙眼的新篇章,为此中国获得了"国际沙眼金质奖章"。之后,国内学者一方面继续沙眼衣原体病原学研究,一方面从临床和防治角度,研究沙眼的致病机理、局部免疫、传播途径、治疗药物和预防措施,并初步探索疫苗的研制,筛查有效药物,实现沙眼防治工作的重大突破[4]。

1987年第一次全国残疾人抽样调查结果显示,沙眼导致视力残疾率为102.01/10万,占各种视力残疾的14.25%(1 611/11 300),沙眼致盲率为46.98/10万,沙眼致低视力率为55.02/10万。根据这次调查结果,沙眼致残率占各种视力残疾的14.25%,居第三位[5]。

自20世纪90年代起,全国防盲技术指导组在全国范围内推广WHO简化分级标准和全方位防治沙眼战略——SAFE战略:提供沙眼倒睫矫正手术(Surgery for Trichiasis,S)、使用适当的抗生素(Antibiotic Treatment,A)、促进个人卫生改善,尤其强调儿童面部清洁(Face Washing,F)、环境改善(Environmental Improvement,E),并结合我国改水改厕、爱国卫生运动等国情,将防沙眼教育写入小学课本,创建了中国特色的SAFE模式,这为消除致盲性沙眼提供了有效可行的方法[6]。

三、加入"视觉2020"行动倡议,提前消灭致盲性沙眼

消除致盲性沙眼是"视觉2020——享有看见的权利"的目标之一[7]。1999年,按WHO的估算,中国有全世界最多的人口和沙眼患者,约占全世界沙眼患者的1/4~1/3,约有600万倒睫患者需要手术,中国的行动对全球消灭致盲性沙眼有重要的意义。2003年中国代表参加了在日内瓦WHO总部召开的"消灭致盲性沙眼全球联盟"会议,会议上WHO对中国的沙眼流行情况的估算结果为活动性沙眼(滤泡性沙眼和浸润性沙眼)患者2 600万例,沙眼性倒睫患者300万例[8]。

2006年第二次全国残疾人抽样调查结果显示,沙眼致视力残疾率为17.62/10万,占各种视力残疾的1.87%。其中沙眼致盲率为7.84/10万,沙眼致低视力病率为10.17/10万[9](图8-1、图8-2)。由于调查结果中没有活动性沙眼相关数据,2004—2007年,研究人员在15个省(自治区、直辖市)开展了中国消灭致盲性沙眼评估,共对59 630名10岁以下儿童沙眼患病情况进行检查,发现滤泡性沙眼阳性率为0.94%,共对82 434名50岁以上成年人沙眼患病情况进行检查,发现沙眼性倒睫阳性率为0.34%。两次调查结果均证明,由于我国政府对改善公共卫生环境和医疗条件的不断努力,我国沙眼的患病率已经从20世纪50年代的城市地区30%,农村地区80%的高患病率大幅下降,不同地区沙眼患病率降至2%~29%[10]。

为进一步巩固沙眼防治成果,全国防盲技术指导组向国家提交《中国实现消灭致盲

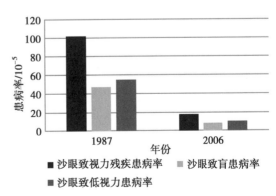

图8-1 1987年和2006年全国沙眼致视力残疾情况比较[11]

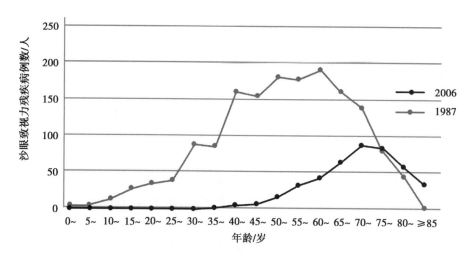

图 8-2　1987 年和 2006 年沙眼致视力残疾病例数的各年龄段分布[11]

性沙眼项目评估书》，并倡导国家卫生行政部门和国际狮子会一起研讨项目计划，并于 2012 年 9 月，在北京启动了"视觉第一中国行动"项目三期——"2016 年前在中国根治致盲性沙眼"项目。该项目由国家主导，国际狮子会资金支持，WHO 防盲人员参与，31 个省（自治区、直辖市）所有的政府、医政管理部门、管理人员、眼科医务人员以及部分残联加入共同推进。"2016 年前在中国根治致盲性沙眼"项目包括对沙眼进行筛查、治疗和评价，在沙眼高发流行疑似区实施沙眼快速评估。项目工作在全国 31 个省（自治区、直辖市）开展，其中在 16 个省份实施沙眼基线评估和患者干预。对 16 个省（自治区、直辖市）130 所小学和 55 679 个村庄对 1~9 岁儿童和 15 岁以上人群开展流行情况调查发现，我国活动性沙眼和沙眼性倒睫患病率分别为 0.196%、0.002%。结果显示，在中国各地，即使是缺水地区也没有再发现沙眼流行的情况，甚至个别高发流行的"口袋"地区，活动性沙眼患病率都低于 5%，沙眼性倒睫低于 0.1%。此外，项目对确诊的 16 名活动性沙眼患者和 1 334 名沙眼性倒睫患者进行了治疗[12,13]。

四、小结

通过我国政府长期的投入与努力，通过防沙眼教育从小抓起，将勤洗手脸、一人一巾等防沙眼知识写入小学教科书，以及改水改厕、全社会爱国卫生运动、环境改善等一系列措施的实施，经济水平和医学水平的提高，国家对农村医疗建设和医疗保险的投入，中国公共卫生条件和医疗条件有了极大的改善，沙眼患者抗生素用药的可及性大大提高，SAFE 战略大力推进实施，中国的沙眼防治工作取得显著成效，在第九次"WHO 消灭致盲性沙眼全球联盟"会议中得到了肯定与赞扬[14]。2015 年 5 月 18 日，在第 68 届 WHA 上，国家卫生和计划生育委员会正式宣布：2014 年中国达到了 WHO 根治致盲性沙眼的要求，提前消灭了致盲性沙眼[13]，沙眼不再是危害我国视觉健康的公共卫生问题。2020 年 2 月 12 日，我国接到

WHO 函告,在对 2019 年 12 月我国提供的文件进行回顾后,WHO 认为沙眼在我国已不再是公共卫生问题,WHO 把全球卫生观察站(Global Health Observatory)页面中的中国沙眼流行状态更改为"已消除作为公共卫生问题"。中国作为占世界总人口近 1/5 的人口大国,提前消灭致盲性沙眼,不仅对中国的卫生与眼健康事业发展与进步具有重大意义,也是世界沙眼防治史上的一项伟大举措,并对在全世界范围内消灭可避免盲具有极大的推动作用和重大贡献。

参 考 文 献

1. 王宁利, 胡爱莲, Hugh R Taylor. 沙眼 [M]. 北京: 人民卫生出版社, 2015: 24-25.

2. 全国沙眼防治规划 (修正草案) 摘要 [J]. 中国医刊, 1959 (3): 1-4.

3. 金秀英. 沙眼衣原体研究历程及进展 [J]. 眼科, 2006, 15 (3): M0145-M0150.

4. Wang N, Deng S, Tian L. A review of trachoma history in China: research, prevention, and control. Science China Life Sciences [J] 2016, 59 (6): 541-547.

5. 全国残疾人抽样调查办公室. 中国 1987 年残疾人抽样调查资料 [Z].

6. 王宁利, 胡爱莲. 我国沙眼防治的启迪与思考 [J]. 中华眼科杂志, 2015 (7): 484-486.

7. 赵家良. "视觉 2020" 行动与我国防盲治盲工作 [J]. 中华眼科杂志, 2002 (10): 4-6.

8. 王宁利, 胡爱莲, Hugh R Taylor. 沙眼 [M]. 北京: 人民卫生出版社, 2015: 37.

9. 第二次全国残疾人抽样调查办公室. 第二次全国残疾人抽样调查资料 [Z]. 中国统计出版社, 2006.

10. 王宁利, 胡爱莲, Hugh R Taylor. 沙眼 [M]. 北京: 人民卫生出版社, 2015: 39.

11. 胡爱莲, 蔡啸谷, 乔利亚, 等. 1987 与 2006 年我国沙眼致视力残疾的对比分析 [J]. 中华眼科杂志, 2015, 51 (10): 768-772.

12. Zhao J, Mariotti S, Resnikoff S, et al. Assessment of trachoma in suspected endemic areas within 16 provinces in mainland China [J]. PLoSNegl Trop Dis, 2019, 13 (1): e0007130.

13. 王宁利, 胡爱莲, Hugh R Taylor. 沙眼 [M]. 北京: 人民卫生出版社, 2015: 49-50.

14. World Health Organization. Report of the Ninth Meeting of the WHO Alliance for the Global Elimination of Blinding Trachoma [C]. 2005: 21.

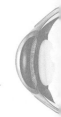

第九章　低视力康复

低视力是"视觉2020"行动倡议中重点工作之一,我国政府承诺:2020年以前,在我国消除包括"低视力"在内的可避免盲。2013年,WHA上通过决议对"视觉2020"行动倡议目标进行调整,提出2014—2019年眼健康全球行动计划,旨在减少作为全球公共卫生问题的可避免视力损害,并使视觉损伤者能够利用康复服务。我国作为加入"视觉2020"行动倡议的成员国之一,积极推动相关工作,制定并实施视力残疾康复政策、计划和方案。

一、中国低视力康复工作的起步

直至20世纪80年代初,低视力康复工作在我国仍是一片空白。1983年北京同仁医院组建了我国第一个低视力门诊,填补了我国低视力康复工作的空白。1986年举办了全国第一个低视力培训班,1986年研制成功第一套国产助视器,1988年出版我国第一部低视力专著《临床低视力学》,2004年主编我国教育部第一部低视力全国高等教材《低视力学》。此外,在全国各地指导建立低视力门诊,低视力康复工作逐渐在全国范围内开展。

二、低视力康复工作的学术交流

自2009年开始,为了解国内外低视力康复工作动态,加强学术交流与合作,分享经验和成果,推动我国低视力康复事业健康发展,国家卫生和计划生育委员会医政医管局、中国残联康复部主办一年一届的"国际低视力康复论坛"。中国视觉障碍资源中心(设于北京同仁医院)致力于视力残疾康复专业人才培养、培训、规范教学、科研开发等工作,于2011年开始承办国际低视力康复论坛,截至2019年,国际低视力康复论坛已圆满举办十届。国内低视力专家、对低视力康复感兴趣的眼科专家,也积极参加国际举办的低视力相关会议,如国际低视力研究与康复协会举办的国际低视力大会等。此外,低视力工作越来越受到眼科专业所重视,在中华医学会眼科学分会年会、中国医师协会眼科医师分会年会,以及多个眼科亚专科的年会中,都设置防盲与低视力专场,方便国内低视力康复专家的交流、学习。

三、我国的低视力康复规划

(一) 低视力或视力残疾康复规划

1991年，我国将低视力康复工作纳入《中国残疾人事业"八五"计划纲要(1991—1995年)》，自此，直到"十三五"规划，中国残疾人联合会都将低视力康复工作作为重点工作之一，通过设立低视力康复部、培训人员、开发供应助视器具、宣传普及知识等措施，培养了大量的低视力康复专业人员，培训了大量儿童低视力家长，已为数十万名低视力者配用助视器，为我国低视力康复工作提供了机构、人员、专业知识和资金等保障。

(二) 重视儿童及青少年低视力康复

2009—2011年，中央财政安排专项补助资金，支持各地实施"中国残联贫困残疾儿童抢救性康复项目"。"0~6岁残疾儿童抢救性康复工程"相继在各省(自治区、直辖市)展开，其中，对视力残疾儿童实施康复训练、验配助视器等成为重点实施项目。2013年，国家下发了《关于印发儿童眼及视力保健等儿童保健相关技术规范的通知》(卫办妇社发〔2013〕26号)，对新生儿出生后定期眼病筛查进行了明确规定。目前，中国正逐步建立起系统化的视觉保健服务，宣传眼病防治知识，及时发现致残因素，尽早干预，减少视力残疾发生，降低经济成本投入，从源头上减少儿童低视力的发生。

四、我国低视力康复工作取得的成绩

(一) 开展多种形式的低视力康复人员培训

由中国残联、国家卫生健康委、全国防盲技术指导组每年组织进行各省(自治区、直辖市)低视力康复骨干人才的培训，各省(自治区、直辖市)相应设置省级、市级培训班，根据各地的实际情况及需求设计培训内容，此外还有不同学会、协会也对眼科医生、康复医生设置低视力康复相关继续教育培训项目，提高低视力筛查诊断水平，加强眼科医疗机构与低视力康复中心的合作，通过技术指导等方式，提高低视力患者的康复服务质量。

(二) 低视力康复网络建设

根据《全国防盲治盲规划(2012—2015年)》(卫医政发〔2012〕52号)要求，省级残疾人康复机构均建立"低视力康复中心"，加强低视力康复中心服务能力建设。建立低视力助视器生产供应服务网络，提高低视力患者的生活质量。在《"十三五"全国眼健康规划(2016—2020年)》中亦要求：三级综合医院眼科和眼科专科医院应普遍提供低视力门诊服务，有条件的医院要开展低视力康复工作。建立眼科医疗机构与低视力康复机构的合作、转诊工作机制。加强眼科医疗机构与疾病预防控制机构或眼病防治机构、低视力康复机构的沟通协作，建立医、防、康复相结合的合作机制。

除此之外，在低视力儿童较集中的盲校，开展低视力分类教学、视功能训练、家长培训，并向社会提供咨询服务；接受培训的家长在家庭对低视力儿童进行视功能训练和助视器使用训练。

（三）国家财政支持的助视器专业验配及康复培训

中国残联在制定的低视力/视力残疾康复规划中要求,中央经费和地方经费应在助视器验配方面提供财政支持,保证验配和培训的免费进行。"十一五"期间为 10 万名贫困低视力者免费配用助视器,培训 3 万名低视力儿童家长。对 3 万名盲人进行定向行走训练[1]。"十二五"期间为 50 万名低视力者免费配用助视器,培训低视力儿童家长 20 万名。对 50 万名盲人进行定向行走训练,配发康复用品用具[2]。根据国务院办公厅发布的《国家残疾预防行动计划(2016—2020 年)》(国办发〔2016〕66 号),至 2020 年,我国将初步建立覆盖城乡的较完善的助视器服务网络,各地形成保障低视力患者基本辅助器具服务的政策体系,验配助视器的服务能力和服务状况都有所提高和改善,有需求的持证残疾人、残疾儿童基本辅助器具适配率达到 80% 以上。

（四）大力支持具有自主产权的助视器研发

助视器是低视力患者补偿和改善功能、提高生存质量、增强社会生活参与能力最直接有效的手段之一。我国自"八五"期间将残疾人辅助器具服务纳入国民经济和社会发展规划以来,取得了显著成效。我国低视力康复工作开展初期,助视器全部依赖进口,直到 1986 年研制成功第一套国产助视器,之后在国家卫生健康委及中国残联的政策支持下,建立了完善的助视器产业发展扶持政策,各省市综合运用财政、税收、金融、土地等手段,引导、鼓励企业、科研机构、高等院校、社会组织等参与助视器研发、生产、流通和适配服务。各种品牌、各种类型、针对低视力患者不同需求的助视器逐步研发、上市,目前,国产助视器工作体系逐步建立,服务体系日趋完善。

（五）相关部门各司其职,形成协调运作机制

各级卫生健康行政部门将低视力康复工作纳入医院眼科工作范畴,明确眼科医生在低视力康复工作中的职责,并对他们进行培训;教育部门积极开展低视力分类教学和家长培训工作;残联做好协调、服务和宣传工作。

五、小结

低视力患者在我国康复领域是一个数量庞大的群体,目前我国低视力康复工作已经取得了一定成绩,尽管当前我国低视力康复现状还存在一定问题,但是可以预见,在国家的统筹规划下,通过全社会尤其是各专业技术人员的共同努力,我国会逐渐形成一个完整、正规的评估、康复系统,帮助低视力患者提高生活质量、参与社会生活。

参 考 文 献

1. 中国残疾人联合会. 视力残疾康复"十一五"实施方案.[EB/OL].(2014-07-25)[2021-07-15]. http://2021old. cdpf. org. cn/ghjh/syfzgh/syw/201407/t20140725_357665. shtml
2. 中国残疾人联合会. 中国残疾人事业"十二五"发展纲要-配套实施方案之三:视力残疾康复"十二五"实施方案.[EB/OL]. (2012-03-06) [2021-07-15]. http://2021old. cdpf. org. cn/ghjh/syfzgh/sew/201203/t20120306_78000. shtml

第十章 眼健康促进

健康促进的意义在于社会各界共同关注健康、支持健康,共同为推动全社会健康水平的提高而努力,形成良好的社会环境和氛围,使大众的健康程度越来越高。健康促进已经成为当前我国应对健康问题的首选策略和核心策略。党的十九大报告中提出要推进健康中国建设,这是党和政府对人民健康的高度重视,也对眼健康促进提出了一个更高的要求。

一、开展眼健康宣传活动

1996 年,原卫生部、教育部、团中央、中国残联等 12 个部委联合发出通知,将每年 6 月 6 日定为"全国爱眼日"[1]。截至 2020 年,我国已经连续举办了 25 个"全国爱眼日"主题活动,围绕加强全民爱眼意识,动员社会各界力量,共同关注眼健康工作。内容涵盖儿童和青少年视力、老年人眼保健、眼外伤、白内障、儿童盲、低视力、白内障、致盲性沙眼、糖尿病视网膜病变、近视等方面。设计"全国爱眼日"的主题与宣传画,通过广播、电视、报纸、网络以及其他新媒体等方式开展眼健康促进教育,普及眼健康知识,增强公众眼病防治意识,降低不同眼病的患病率和提高知晓率,在全社会营造积极参与眼病防治工作的良好舆论氛围。

2005 年,"3·15"晚会上通过"看不到光,我很可怜"的案例,呼吁全社会人士关注早产儿过度吸氧的危害及早产儿视网膜病变的防治。近年来,随着我国对产科、儿科和眼科等医务人员进行早产儿抢救治疗用氧和视网膜病变的预防、诊断、治疗方面的培训,建立医疗机构间的转诊制度,开展早产儿视网膜病变的远程诊断筛查,组织成立儿童保健技术指导组,开展早产儿医疗保健业务培训和早产儿健康教育工作[2],推广相关适宜技术,发放相关健康教育材料,早产儿视网膜病变发病率和重症率逐年下降。如深圳市 2008 年早产儿视网膜病变发病率、重症率为 14.64%、6.52%,2013 年则降至 11.47%、4.26%,较 20 世纪 90 年代有了大幅下降[3]。

利用"联合国糖尿病日"等主题宣传日活动、健康知识传播激励计划和日常科普宣传活动,组织安排眼科与内分泌科医务人员走进社区、养老院、离退休干部中心等,推动糖尿病视网膜病变防治工作"关口前移",在基层医疗卫生机构、内分泌科和眼科之间构建分级诊疗服务模式,通过专家在公共媒体或网络上对糖尿病及糖尿病视网膜病变的宣传教育、义诊筛查、咨询、科普大讲堂、张贴宣传海报、发放宣传手册等方式,推广宣传糖尿病防治指南,广泛传播糖尿病及糖尿病眼病等并发症防治知识,使公众对糖尿病及糖尿病视网膜病变的知晓率达到 76.7%[4],对糖尿病患者能够及时有效地就医具有积极推动作用,糖尿病视网膜病变的早期发现、早期诊断率也随之提高。

在全国范围内开展"儿童青少年预防近视"系列主题宣传活动。目前,有关部门(教育部、国家卫生健康委、体育总局、财政部、人力资源社会保障部、市场监管总局、国家新闻出版署、国家广电总局)、学校、医疗卫生机构、家庭、学生等各方面共同努力,共同关心、支持、保护儿童青少年视力的工作。全社会行动起来,通过媒体传播、召开工作研讨会、宣传栏张贴海报、家长会、家长信等多种形式进行广泛的宣传,视力筛查、建立视觉健康档案,让孩子参与到爱眼护眼的漫画制作中,通过画作展现对爱眼护眼的认识,让孩子自觉主动呵护好自己的眼睛。在全社会营造了儿童青少年视力保护"政府主导、部门配合、专家指导、学校教育、家庭关注"的良好氛围。

2008 年 3 月 6 日是第一个"世界青光眼日",迄今为止已连续举办了十一次宣传活动。"世界青光眼日"是由世界青光眼联合会和世界青光眼患者联合会共同发起的一项全球性行动,旨在提高青光眼的知晓率,其目标为到 2020 年,青光眼的未诊断率从 50% 降低到 20% 以下[5]。近年来,随着政府部门、眼科医生及眼保健专业人员等通过媒体宣传、现场义诊咨询、青光眼知识讲座、患者交流会等形式的宣传,目前,开角型青光眼的检出率则从 10% 上升到 40%[6]。

每年十月份的第 2 个星期四是"世界视觉日",自 2000 年开始,它成为"视觉 2020"的主要宣传活动,是由 WHO 主导,结合国际防盲协会、国际狮子会、国际奥比斯等全球多个国际志愿机构共同订立的全球医疗公益行动。我国的多个志愿机构通过宣传讲座、义诊咨询、视力筛查、社区教育活动、回收旧眼镜等宣传途径,提高公众对盲和视力损害的重视,向公众宣传盲的预防知识和"视觉 2020"行动倡议。

二、国家大力弘扬眼科医学人文精神

眼科是整个临床医疗体系中非常重要的一部分。在眼健康工作中,眼科医务工作者不仅要做好疾病的临床诊断与治疗,还需要关注防盲治盲等公共卫生与眼病防治工作。国家通过大力弘扬"大医精诚、救死扶伤"的优良传统,鼓励眼科医务人员和基层医疗卫生工作者深入贫困地区为贫困群众解除眼病。此外,眼科医务人员也通过广播、报刊、电视、网络等多种形式开展眼健康宣教工作,促进全社会重视眼病防治工作,提高眼科公共卫生和眼病预防水平,有效地提高了眼科疾病的防控能力,使得"视觉 2020,享有看见的权利"深入每一个人的心中。为表彰眼科医务人员在防盲事业上所作出的杰出贡献,亚太眼科学会在 2005—2019 年共为 42 位中国眼科医务工作者颁发了防盲杰出服务奖,中华医学会眼科学分会于 2014 年、2016 年共为 6 位眼科医务工作者颁发了防盲杰出贡献奖。

参 考 文 献

1. 国家卫生健康委员会. 全国爱眼日 [EB/OL].[2020-06-17]. http://www. nhc. gov. cn/jnr/qgayrjrjj/qgayr_lmtt. shtml

2. 陈亦棋, 祝晨婷, 沈丽君, 等. 早产儿视网膜病变远程筛查的有效性评估 [J]. 中华眼底病杂志, 2017, 33 (6): 633-634.

3. 深圳市早产儿视网膜病变协作组. 深圳地区早产儿视网膜病变 10 年发病情况分析 [J]. 中华眼底病杂志, 2014, 30 (1): 12-16.

4. Wang, D, Ding X, He M, et al. Use of eye care services among diabetic patients in urban and rural China [J]. Ophthalmology, 2010, 117 (9): 1755-1762.

5. 国家卫生健康委员会. 世界青光眼日 [EB/OL].(2014-03-04)[2020-06-17]. http://www. nhc. gov. cn/jnr/qgyjrjj/201403/238de4b376c74d699574f4bb3d7a489f. shtml.

6. 李惠民. 湘潭县农村原发性青光眼致盲率调查 [J]. 湖南医学, 1986 (3): 158.

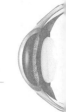

第十一章　我国眼库发展

一、概况

眼库是指在医疗机构内设置，从事公民逝世后捐献角膜的获取转运、保存处理、质量评估和启动分配的组织或机构。我国发展比较早的眼库有北京同仁眼库、河南省眼科研究所眼库、广东省眼库和山东省眼库等。1997年国际眼库联合会将北京同仁眼库、上海眼耳鼻喉医院眼库、山东省眼科研究所眼库接纳为正式会员单位。眼库的发展水平与角膜盲患者是否可以得到有效治疗密切相关。

二、我国眼库的现状与问题

调查显示，全国共有78家眼库，与发达国家相比，我国眼库存在角膜供体来源不足及后续角膜预处理水平低等问题。其中捐献角膜数量少是影响我国眼库发展及可治疗角膜盲患者得不到有效治疗的根本原因。

三、工作进展

针对我国眼库发展现状与问题，2017年起，全国防盲技术指导组办公室在国家卫生健康委医政医管局的指导下，推动开展相关工作。

（一）对眼库情况进行全面调查，了解眼库基本情况。目前我国正在运行的眼库有14家，每年处理眼球约3 500个，每年使用角膜2 800片。

（二）2018年全国防盲技术指导组成立眼库管理专家委员会，以推动我国眼库事业发展、提高眼库管理和质量水平为目标，主要开展以下工作：编订眼库技术标准，建立眼库管理规范，推动眼库医生和技术人员的培训；建立国家级捐献网上注册信息登记系统；扩大角膜捐献的公众认知，提高公民捐献的合作意识；建立眼库质量控制体系等。

（三）组织制定眼库管理规范等文件。为规范眼库建设，明确眼库管理要求，保障捐献角膜质量和医疗安全,维护人民群众健康权益,在国家卫生健康行政部门的指导下,全国防盲技术指导组眼库专家委员会制定了《眼库管理规范》《眼库操作技术指南》和《眼库质量管理与控制指标》,详细规范了眼库管理和技术操作的各个环节,并制定了相关质量控制指标。

(四)建立中国人体角膜分配与共享系统。该系统遵循人体角膜分配与共享应当符合医疗需要,遵循公平、公正和公开的原则,对捐献角膜进行全过程管理,公平分配、合理使用角膜,按照眼库所属移植医院等待名单、眼库服务区域内的移植医院等待名单、省级等待名单、全国等待名单四个层级逐级进行分配与共享。角膜分配系统负责执行角膜分配与共享政策。角膜必须通过角膜分配系统进行分配与共享。任何机构、组织和个人不得在角膜分配系统外擅自分配角膜。该系统于2019年10月起在全国10个省(自治区、直辖市)开始试点。

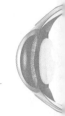

第十二章　中国防盲公益活动国际化

随着我国眼科诊疗水平的提高,中国的防盲公益活动不仅在国内广泛开展,也走出中国、走向国际。

2003 年,全国防盲技术指导组整合全国防盲资源,启动了集流行病学调查、专业培训、医疗和健康教育为一体的"光明行"活动,医疗队足迹遍及全国老少边穷及高原地区,目前已帮助国内 4 万余名白内障患者重见光明。

2008 年"光明行"首次跨出国门,赴邻邦朝鲜、柬埔寨进行活动,此后医疗队还先后抵达亚太地区的蒙古、老挝、越南、孟加拉国、巴基斯坦等国家及地区,开展公益活动。2010 年"光明行"活动走入非洲,先后在津巴布韦、马拉维、赞比亚和莫桑比克等开展白内障复明活动。2012 年 7 月,在中非合作论坛第五届部长级会议上,我国政府宣布继续深化中非务实合作的新举措,其中包括继续扩大对非援助,继续开展"光明行"活动,为非洲白内障患者提供免费治疗。2015 年 12 月,习近平总书记在中非合作论坛约翰内斯堡峰会开幕式上致辞时将"中非公共卫生合作计划"作为未来三年同非方重点实施的"十大合作计划"之一予以提出。

2015 年,原国家卫生计生委出台的《国家卫生计生委关于推进"一带一路"卫生交流合作三年实施方案(2015—2017)》(国卫办国际函〔2015〕866 号)中也明确将开展"光明行"眼科义诊活动列为卫生发展援助的重要内容之一。为进一步推进并落实我国的国际卫生交流合作方案,全国各省(自治区、直辖市)先后派遣医疗队赴友好国家开展"光明行"活动——白内障复明手术。至今,中国已在朝鲜、越南、老挝、柬埔寨、缅甸、蒙古、泰国、孟加拉国、巴基斯坦、也门、巴哈马、津巴布韦、马拉维、赞比亚、莫桑比克、布隆迪、毛里塔尼亚、博茨瓦纳、牙买加、安提瓜和巴布达、斯里兰卡、喀麦隆、科摩罗、刚果(布)、多哥、贝宁、苏丹、塞内加尔、哈萨克斯坦、乍得、吉布提、乌兹别克斯坦、斐济、汤加、瓦努阿图、萨摩亚、巴布亚新几内亚、密克罗尼西亚、库克群岛、纽埃、纳米比亚、塞拉利昂等 40 多个国家开展"光明行"活动,其中十个国家是多次活动,使数万名白内障患者重见光明。

"光明行"不仅为当地人民免费实施白内障复明手术,捐赠先进眼科手术设备和器械药品,还为学生进行了视力筛查、捐赠眼镜,开展复杂性眼底病和青光眼手术。在当地开展学术讲座、临床带教,与相关国家建立了"眼科合作中心",利用互联网进行眼病的远程会诊,拓展多种形式技术交流与合作。同时关注人才培养,组织当地医生赴中国培训。

中国的防盲公益事业国际化,为被援助国家人民带去了光明,充分彰显了我国在为构建人类命运共同体及在一带一路沿线国家中的作为与贡献,也成为中国外交的重要力量,进一步推进了卫生国际交流合作。

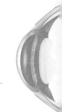

第十三章　眼科自主研发能力提升

眼科作为一门多知识体系综合交叉性学科,眼病的诊断和治疗高度依赖于各种设备,眼科设备的优劣,在一定程度上决定了诊治水平的高低。随着现代高科技水平的发展,眼科诊疗设备的临床实用性、安全性、智能性、更新速度都飞速发展,并对眼科疾患的防治、医疗质量的保障起着重要的作用。

一、眼科医疗产品与设备的研发和应用

(一)眼科医疗产品的需求分析

眼科医疗产品一般分为眼科设备、眼科耗材、眼科药物、视光产品四部分。70% 的眼病治疗以手术为主,对器械依赖性较高。2017 年,全球眼科医疗器械与耗材销售规模 277 亿美元,占全部医疗器械与耗材总销售规模的 6.8%,是全球第五大医疗器械领域。预测 2024 年销售规模将达 422 亿美元,年均复合增长率为 6.2%,高于医疗器械与耗材行业的整体值 5.6%,届时销售规模占比将增加至 7.1%。我国眼用药市场规模已超 150 亿元,创新靶点、创新剂型等眼科用药的推出有力拉动了市场的增长。2017 年中国眼镜零售市场规模 730 亿元,预计 2020 年中国眼镜行业市场规模将进一步扩大,市场规模将达 850 亿元。

(二)国产眼科医疗产品的发展概况

国内前 8 大眼科医疗产品公司销售规模占据了全国市场的 73.3%,其中外资品牌占据了近 50%。国内生产企业在技术、高端材料及研发资金等方面与外企存在较大差距,普遍规模不大,还有巨大的进口替代空间。

随着我国医疗保障制度日趋完善,医疗改革对基层医疗单位防盲的投入逐年增加,加大适宜基层使用的眼科诊疗设备的研发力度、满足基层眼健康服务需求对国家医疗保健卫生全方面发展至关重要。科技部科研立项数据检索结果显示,“十二五”和“十三五”期间,国家支持对眼科常见病和多发病的小型移动式医疗服务装备、高值耗材、创新药物进行了重点研究开发,累计投资国家级课题资金 9 000 余万元。

近年来,我国眼科资源总量大幅增加,但是由于我国幅员辽阔,仍然存在资源分布不均的问题。尤其是在边远贫困地区,眼科资源的可及性较差,眼科基本服务不完善。尽管不同

医疗机构、社会团体组织的光明行和义诊为这些地区的眼疾患者带来了希望,但是传统眼科检查和治疗设备体积庞大,限制了其运输及在防盲义诊过程中的使用。近年来,多个厂家推出了多款便携式检查设备,如:便携式验光仪、便携式裂隙灯、便携式检眼镜等检查设备,这些设备在防盲领域的应用,提高了眼病的检出率和准确率,为后续对患者提供有效的治疗提供了基础。除了便携式检查设备,一些便携式的治疗设备也被陆续推出,如:便携式超声乳化仪、便携式手术显微镜。

由于眼科疾病比较复杂,故眼科设备产品种类也较多,常用的眼病专科设备有视力表、裂隙灯、直接/间接检眼镜、眼压计、验光仪、房角镜、三面镜、视野计、眼科用 A/B 超声诊断仪、眼科超声生物显微镜(UBM)、角膜曲率计、角膜内皮细胞计数仪、眼科电生理仪、光学相干断层扫描仪(OCT)、角膜地形图仪、视网膜荧光眼底造影机、YAG 激光仪、光凝激光设备、氩离子激光机、手术显微镜、白内障超声乳化机、玻璃体切割机视网膜冷冻仪等。

其中常用眼科诊断类设备已经基本实现了国产化,产品的市场占有率逐年提高,眼科超声、OCT、UBM 等产品已经开始进入国际市场。在眼科治疗类设备方面,医生更加注重产品的安全性和稳定性,因此对产品的技术含量和质量水平有着更高的要求。国内生产企业在技术、高端材料及研发资金等方面与外企存在较大差距,普遍规模不大。特别是白内障、近视治疗两大细分行业市场依旧被国外企业垄断。

国内眼科药品市场集中度高,眼科制药三大国际巨头占比约为 45.12%;国内龙头企业占比 14.03%。国内龙头企业近五年在眼底抗新生血管、眼干燥症治疗创新药的研制方面取得了长足的进步,市场占有率呈逐年提升的态势。

人工晶体是白内障手术的主要耗材,我国市场规模约 100 亿元。近五年国产品牌在软式(可折叠)人工晶状体方面取得了突破,市场占有率已提升至 15% 左右。角膜塑形镜作为控制青少年近视进展的方法,近年来呈爆发性增长态势。2018 年市场规模约 51 亿元,而2014 年仅为 15.3 亿元,每年均保持 30% 左右的快速增长,国内企业目前市场占有率约为20%。

矫正屈光不正用的框架眼镜是视光产品的最主要类别。通常在欧美国家,框架眼镜市场是眼科医疗市场的一部分,属于医疗产品;在国内,由于历史沿革的原因,框架眼镜属于消费品市场。由于市场管理部门与国外不同,造成框架眼镜市场产品良莠不齐。虽然经过长时间的行业发展,国内市场仍然被国外公司垄断。近年来国内企业在镜片精密验配及加工、镜框个性化定制等领域取得了技术突破。

二、远程眼科与人工智能的研发与应用

随着信息技术和互联网的飞速发展,患者可以获得高质量的远程医疗服务。为了规范发展"互联网 +"医疗健康,推进远程医疗工作,为人民群众提供更加便利的医疗服务,2018 年 9 月 14 日国家卫生健康委与国家中医药管理局发布了《关于印发互联网诊疗管理办法(试行)等 3 个文件的通知》(国卫医发〔2018〕25 号),共同制定了《互联网诊疗管理办法(试行)》《互联网医院管理办法(试行)》《远程医疗服务管理规范(试行)》3 个文件。文件

的出台旨在进一步规范互联网的诊疗行为,发挥远程医疗服务的积极作用,提高医疗服务的效率。

远程医疗技术普及推广很快,对平衡医疗资源发挥了非常大的作用。不仅全国所有三甲医院都开通了远程医疗服务,而且我国已实现所有国家级贫困县县医院远程医疗全覆盖。2019 年 7 月 9 日,国家卫生健康委召开新闻发布会表示,截至 2018 年底,三级医院已派出超过 6 万人次医务人员参与贫困县县级医院管理和诊疗工作,门诊诊疗人次超过 3 000 万,管理出院患者超过 300 万,住院手术超过 50 万台。通过派驻人员的传、帮、带,帮助县医院新建临床专科 5 900 个,开展新技术、新项目超过 3.8 万项。已有超过 400 家贫困县医院成为二级甲等医院,30 余家贫困县医院达到三级医院水平。三级医院优质医疗服务有效下沉,贫困县县医院服务能力和管理水平明显提升。

而以图像检查为主要辅助诊断手段的眼科在远程医疗的发展中具有巨大优势,是最适合远程医疗的学科之一。眼科远程医疗的开展将有助于下沉优秀医疗资源,解决眼科医疗资源分布不均的难题。有研究表明,远程眼科在糖尿病视网膜病变、青光眼等慢性眼病的筛查中更具成本效益[1]。我国已经开发了多个眼科远程医疗系统,并取得了良好的效果,通过在三级医院成立远程眼科会诊中心与基层医院建立了协同医疗模式,这为青光眼筛查和诊断提供了一种有效而便捷的手段[2]。

人工智能的迅速发展也为辅助眼科诊疗和疾病预测带来了新的突破口。2017 年 11 月 15 日,科技部召开新一代人工智能发展规划暨重大科技项目启动会,介绍了新一代人工智能发展规划实施的组织推进机制,宣布成立新一代人工智能发展规划推进办公室;介绍了新一代人工智能发展规划部署实施的前期准备,强调规划实施要构建开放协同的人工智能科技创新体系;宣布首批国家新一代人工智能开放创新平台名单,其中包括了医疗影像国家新一代人工智能开放创新平台。

2017 年 12 月,原国家卫生计生委印发《医院信息化建设应用技术指引》(国卫办规划函〔2017〕1232 号),提出人工智能在健康医疗服务、医疗智能应用和医院智能管理等方面的具体应用技术要求。2018 年 4 月,国家卫生健康委印发《全国医院信息化建设标准与规范(试行)》(国卫办规划发〔2018〕4 号),对医院开展疾病风险预测、医学影像辅助诊断、临床辅助诊疗、智能健康管理、医院智能管理、虚拟助理等人工智能应用提出具体要求。

目前人工智能眼科图像诊断已经应用于多种致盲性眼病的诊断,如:白内障、青光眼、糖尿病视网膜病变、年龄相关性黄斑变性等。以糖尿病视网膜病变为例,根据 2018 年国际糖尿病联盟公布的数据,我国约 5 亿人处于糖尿病前期,糖尿病患者约有 1.1 亿人,糖尿病视网膜病变患者约有 3 000 万[3]。人工智能在糖尿病视网膜病变早期筛查和诊断上具有较高的准确率。近年来,众多企业、科研机构均进行了关于此方面的研究,多家公司研发了眼底图像质量评估、糖尿病视网膜病变严重程度分级、病灶位置检测等智能算法,最终自动生成结构化筛查报告,为患者提供转诊建议。在青光眼领域,据 2011 年统计数据显示,我国 40 岁以上人群的青光眼患病率为 2.6%,致盲率为 30%。在我国若对所有患者进行治疗,估计直接花费可达 150 亿~180 亿美元[4,5]。目前,由我国研究团队研发的可以自动检测眼底图像的青光眼性视神经改变的深度学习算法[6]已经实现了人工智能识别过程的可视化,并作为"来自中国真实世界的多中心研究"获得了眼视光学在线杂志 OPTOMERTY TIMES 的专题报道;此外,该团队还与互联网公司合作,共同研发了国内首款青光眼可视化筛查产品。目前,人工智能不仅能够用于诊断常见致盲性眼病,还能够对儿童近视的发展进行预测[7]。

在 2020 年 5 月举行的健康医疗人工智能焦点组第九次会议中,来自北京研究团队的 2 份关于"人工智能影像技术在眼底疾病筛查"的应用标准及技术要求全部被健康医疗人工智能焦点组采纳[8,9]。这意味着我国在眼底疾病人工智能影像筛查方面所做的工作已转化为健康医疗人工智能方面的国际标准,未来会成为 WHO 及联合国国际电信联盟在人工智能医疗领域的推荐标准,并被各国药监机构以及相关医疗企业参考。相信在不远的未来,随着人工智能的不断发展和相关政策的进一步完善,人工智能会带来从筛查到诊断的全面革新,为整个眼科学的发展注入新的活力。

参 考 文 献

1. Sharafeldin N, Kawaguchi A, Sundaram A, et al. Review of economic evaluations of teleophthalmology as a screening strategy for chronic eye disease in adults [J]. Br J Ophthalmol, 2018, 102 (11): 1485-1491.

2. 张莉, 徐捷, 曹凯, 等. 远程眼科会诊对青光眼检出效果影响的研究 [J]. 中华眼科医学杂志 (电子版), 2019 (4): 206-211.

3. International Diabetes Federation. IDF Diabetes Atlas.[EB/OL].[2020-06-02]. http://www. diabetesatlas. org/.

4. Rein D, Zhang P, Wirth K, et al. The economic burden of major adult visual disorders in the united states [J]. Archives of Ophthalmology, 2006, 124 (12): 1754-1760.

5. Liang Y, Friedman D, Zhou Q, et al. Prevalence of Primary Open Angle Glaucoma in a Rural Adult Chinese Population: The Handan Eye Study [J]. Investigative Ophthalmology & Visual Science, 2011, 52 (11): 8250-8257.

6. Liu H, Li L, Wormstone I, et al. Development and Validation of a Deep Learning System to Detect Glaucomatous Optic Neuropathy Using Fundus Photographs [J]. JAMA Ophthalmology, 2019, 137 (12): 1353-1360.

7. Lin H, Long E, Ding X, et al. Prediction of myopia development among Chinese school-aged children using refraction data from electronic medical records: A retrospective, multicentre machine learning study [J]. Plos Med, 2018, 15 (11): 167-175.

8. Wu J, Zhu Y, Zhang Y, et al. Evaluation method and index of artificial intelligence glaucoma assisted screening system based on fundus image [Z]. ITU-T Focus Group on AI for Health, INTERNATIONAL TELECOMMUNICATION UNION. 2020.

9. Wu J, Zhu Y, Zhang Y, et al. Data set construction and annotation of artificial intelligence assisted screening system based on fundus image [Z]. ITU-T Focus Group on AI for Health, INTERNATIONAL TELECOM-MUNICATION UNION. 2020.

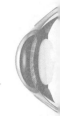

第十四章　我国眼健康面临的挑战

眼病流行病学研究是开展防盲治盲的基础性工作之一。近年来,我国开展了多个大型眼病流行病学调查,如广州荔湾眼病研究、开滦眼病研究、北京眼病研究、邯郸眼病研究[1-4]等,为我国眼健康现状摸底提供了大量可靠的证据。各大眼病流行病学调查的数据,以及近年来我国开展的眼病疾病负担研究[5]显示,我国的眼病负担稳中有变。

一、屈光不正和白内障疾病负担最重

具体来看,从 1990 年到 2020 年[5],中国最主要的眼病负担一直是屈光不正,且无论在哪个年龄段屈光不正均是导致视力损伤的主要原因。屈光不正的年龄标准化患病率每年都远高于其他眼病。第二位的疾病负担是白内障(图 14-1,图 14-2)。屈光不正和白内障是我国亟待解决的最主要的眼健康负担。

二、患病率稳中有降,但患病人数上升

从患病率来看,各个年龄层每种眼病的患病情况仍基本维持稳定,各类眼病的排名如下:屈光不正居第一位,白内障居第二位。同时我们可以看到一个很明显的趋势:随着我国社会老龄化的不断加重,尽管屈光不正和白内障的年龄标准化患病率从 1990 年到 2020 年并未明显上升,处在基本稳定的状态,但是由于人口总数增加和人口老龄化,屈光不正和白内障的患病人数却在大大增加。

三、黄斑病变有抬头趋势

另外值得注意的是:在 2005 年以前,我国青光眼的患病人数高于黄斑病变,而在 2005 年以后,黄斑病变的患病人数开始逐年上升并反超青光眼。从年龄标准化患病率的角度来看,黄斑病变的患病人数从 2000 年开始就已经超过青光眼。黄斑病变是眼底疾病,与人们的生活水平、生活方式密切相关,眼底疾病的防控亟需引起政府和人们的重视。

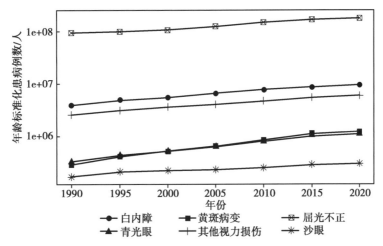

图 14-1　1990 年至 2020 年中国各类主要眼病的患病人数

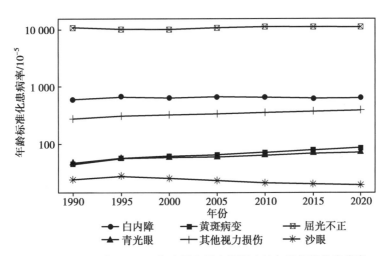

图 14-2　1990 年至 2020 年中国各类主要眼病的年龄标准化患病率

四、中老年人群疾病负担增长最重

从 1990 年到 2015 年，我国 0 至 14 岁人群无论在眼病患病人数方面还是在因视力损伤导致的健康寿命损失方面，均有较大幅度的降低（图 14-3）；而在 15 岁及以上人群中，这两项指标均有较大幅度的增长。尤其是 50 岁及以上人群中，增长幅度极其显著。

1990 年，50 岁及以上人群中的青光眼患病率居第四位，黄斑变性排名居第五位；而到 2015 年，在 50 岁及以上人群中，黄斑变性的患病率排名上升到第四位，青光眼在这个年龄段中排名下降到第五位。

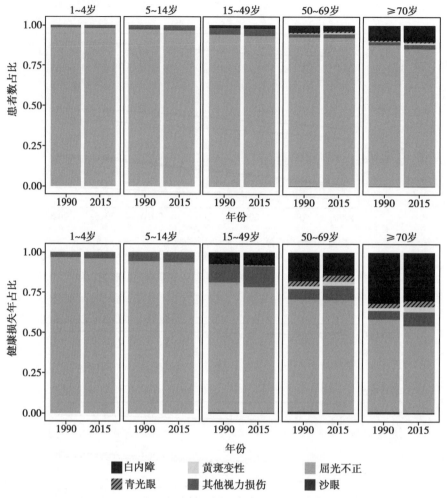

图 14-3 1990 年至 2015 年中国各年龄组人群的
眼病患病人数及视力损伤所致的健康寿命损失年总量

综上,中国眼健康目前所面临的最大的挑战是人口增多,更是老龄化的不断加剧。截至 2019 年,我国 60 岁以上人口已达到 25 388 万人,占全国总人口的 18.1%,并且老龄人口仍在不断增多。老年人数量的增加意味着年龄相关性眼病的患者数量在不断增加,包括屈光不正和白内障,而这两类眼病正是我国的主要眼病负担。此外,常见的主要致盲性眼病,包括青光眼、黄斑病变等眼底疾病,也都是年龄相关性眼病,在老年人群中的患病率远高于年轻人,这些仍是我国眼健康工作面临的挑战和未来眼健康工作的重点。

———————————— 参 考 文 献 ————————————

1. Yan Y, Wang Y, Yang Y, et al. Ten-year progression of myopic maculopathy: the Beijing Eye Study 2001-2011 [J]. Ophthalmology, 2018, 125 (8): 1253-1263.

2. Wang L, Zhao Y, Han X, et al. Five-year visual outcome among people with correctable visual impairment: the Liwan Eye Study [J]. Clin Exp Ophthalmol, 2018, 46 (5): 462-467.

3. Wang Q, Wang Y, Wu S, et al. Ocular axial length and diabetic retinopathy: the Kailuan Eye Study [J]. Invest Ophthalmol Vis Sci, 2019, 60 (10): 3689-3695.

4. Cao K, Hao J, Zhang Y, et al. Design, methodology, and preliminary results of the follow-up of a population-based cohort study in rural area of northern China: Handan Eye Study [J]. Chin Med J (Engl), 2019, 132 (18): 2157-2167.

5. Wang B, Congdon N, Bourne R, et al. Burden of vision loss associated with eye disease in China 1990-2020: findings from the Global Burden of Disease Study 2015 [J]. Br J Ophthalmol, 2018, 102 (2): 220-224.

结 束 语

随着生活方式的改变、社会发展及人口老龄化,我国眼科疾病谱已发生了重大变化。我们应该根据国家《"健康中国 2030"规划纲要》,将眼健康纳入大健康,制定我国眼健康规划。此外,在"十四五"全国眼健康规划中,要从关注常见致盲性眼病转变,将重点放在角膜病、青光眼、代谢相关性眼病以及年龄相关性眼病等重大致盲性眼病。转变我国眼科资源配置的地区不平衡现状,促进平衡发展,将致盲性眼病的治疗转向疾病的防控,特别要关注主要致盲性眼病防治技术下沉,加强基层眼科和眼科队伍建设,继续完善我国三级防盲体系的建设。同时,依托中国县级医院眼科团队培训项目等健康扶贫项目,将眼科服务能力建设与国家扶贫攻坚工作结合,通过健康扶贫促进健康中国的发展。

根据国情制定白内障手术防治指标,根据社会经济发展水平,适度放宽适应证。此外,对于白内障复明手术的评价,既要考虑数量,更要评价质量,关注世界卫生组织最新提出的有效白内障手术覆盖率这一指标。儿童青少年近视已成为我国视力损伤的主要原因,要坚决贯彻执行国家关于近视防控的实施方案,实现我国儿童青少年近视防控的目标,同时关注世界卫生组织最新提出的有效屈光不正校正覆盖率这一指标。

此外,在常用眼科设备和技术方面,要大力推动国产化,彻底改变严重依赖进口设备和技术的现状。在共性技术、"卡脖子"技术方面,有所突破。要继续推进可防可控致盲性眼病适宜技术的培训和推广,将关口前移减少发病率,增加控制效果。在技术成熟时,应推广基于人工智能技术的眼病筛查,做到致盲性眼病的早发现早治疗,在我国经济条件允许的前提下,考虑到系统性疾病所导致的眼病患者人数呈上升趋势,尽可能争取把常见致盲性眼病的筛查纳入慢性病管理体系之中。通过科学普及工作,增强民众对眼病防治基本知识的了解,提高知晓率,增强民众致盲性眼病防控意识,将科普工作纳入国家眼健康规划和国家健康大科普计划中。

眼科工作者要在国家卫生健康委的领导下,形成两个合作环,在国际上,与世界卫生组织、国际防盲协会、国际眼科理事会等机构紧密合作,与全球共享中国眼健康工作经验和成果。在国内,与中华预防医学会、中华医学会眼科学分会等各个学会合作,在国内学术团队和医疗单位的支持下,共同为构建光明中国而努力。

致　谢

党和政府长期以来十分重视眼健康工作,正是在国家卫生健康委的领导和支持下,在眼健康政策的引导下,我国眼健康工作才取得长足的进展。在此,特别感谢国家卫生健康委医政医管局长期以来对防盲和眼健康工作的指导以及对本白皮书的撰写和发布进行的指导。此外,十分感谢世界卫生组织对中国防盲和眼健康工作的长期支持以及提供技术指导,包括沙眼防治、开展视中三期评估、进行人员培训等各方面的大力支持。另外,感谢国际防盲协会长期以来对中国防盲工作的支持,以及在合作过程中为中国推广适宜防盲技术作出的重要贡献。最后,诚挚地感谢全国眼科同仁在我国眼健康工作中所做的共同努力以及本白皮书成书过程中的大力支持。

Contents

Chapter Ⅰ　Eye Health Service System ··· 59

　　　Ⅰ. Improvement of eye health system in China under the principle
　　　　 of "led by government and participated by all parties" ·························59

　　　Ⅱ. Eye Health Plan ·· 60

　　　Ⅲ. Changes in eye health policies ·· 62

Chapter Ⅱ　Eye Disease Prevention and Treatment Work
　　　　　　 Pattern with Chinese Characteristics ······················· 65

　　　Ⅰ. Government coordination and policy guidance ······························ 65

　　　Ⅱ. Technical support from academic bodies ································· 66

　　　Ⅲ. Active participation of private hospitals and social organizations ···············69

Chapter Ⅲ　Progress under "VISION 2020" Initiative ················· 72

　　　Ⅰ. "VISION 2020" initiative ··· 72

　　　Ⅱ. "VISION 2020" in China ·· 73

　　　Ⅲ. Progress in eliminating avoidable blindness ··························· 74

Chapter Ⅳ　Ophthalmic Resources ··· 79

　　　Ⅰ. Increase of the number of county-level ophthalmology institutions,
　　　　 and strengthening of service capabilities ································· 79

　　　Ⅱ. Growing of ophthalmic personnel team ································· 80

　　　Ⅲ. Gradual improvement of equipping of ophthalmic equipment ·············· 83

Chapter Ⅴ　Significant Reduction of Blindness and Visual
　　　　　　 Impairment ··· 85

Chapter Ⅵ　Changes in Spectrum of Major Blinding Eye
　　　　　　 Diseases ··· 87

Ⅰ. Cataract ································ 87

Ⅱ. Keratopathy ································ 87

Ⅲ. Retinal diseases such as maculopathy and diabetic retinopathy ············· 88

Ⅳ. Refractive error ································ 89

Ⅴ. Glaucoma ································ 89

Ⅵ. Amblyopia ································ 90

Chapter Ⅶ Prevention and Control of Myopia ································ 92

Ⅰ. Current situation of myopia in children and adolescents ············· 92

Ⅱ. National strategy for prevention and control of myopia ············· 93

Ⅲ. Comprehensive prevention and control measures ············· 95

Chapter Ⅷ Elimination of Blinding Trachoma ································ 97

Ⅰ. High prevalence of trachoma in the 1950s ············· 97

Ⅱ. Comprehensive prevention and treatment, scientific research, and remarkable progress ································ 97

Ⅲ. Achieving the goal of eliminating blinding trachoma in advance under the "VISION 2020" initiative ································ 99

Ⅳ. Summary ································ 101

Chapter Ⅸ Low Vision Rehabilitation ································ 103

Ⅰ. Initiation of low vision rehabilitation work in China ············· 103

Ⅱ. Academic exchange in low vision rehabilitation ············· 103

Ⅲ. Low Vision Rehabilitation Plan ································ 104

Ⅳ. Achievements in low vision rehabilitation in China ············· 105

Ⅴ. Summary ································ 107

Chapter Ⅹ Promotion of Eye Health ································ 108

Ⅰ. Eye health promotion activities ································ 108

Ⅱ. Vigorous promotion of medical humanistic spirit ············· 110

Chapter Ⅺ Development of Eye Banks in China ································ 112

Ⅰ. Overview ································ 112

Ⅱ. Current situation of and problems faced by eye banks in China ············· 112

Ⅲ. Progress ································ 112

Chapter XII   Internationalization of Public Welfare Activities in
              Blindness Prevention in China ·················114

Chapter XIII Improvement of Independent Research and
              Development Ability ···················116

        I . Research & development and application of ophthalmic medical
            products and equipment··················116
        II . Research & development and application of remote ophthalmology
            and artificial intelligence (AI)···············118

Chapter XIV   Eye Health Challenges in China ············ 122

        I . Refractive error and cataract ranked top 2 in terms of disease
            burden ·····························122
        II . The prevalence steadily declined, but the number affected has
            increased ··························· 122
        III. The maculopathy is on the rise··············· 123
        IV. The burden of eye disease has increased the most among the
            middle-aged and elderly population ············ 124

Afterword ······························· 126

Acknowledgements ····················· 128

Chapter I Eye Health Service System

I. Improvement of eye health system in China under the principle of "led by government and participated by all parties"

The Chinese government attaches great importance to the prevention and treatment of blindness and has developed the blindness prevention and treatment plan or eye health plan every five years since the 7th 5-Year National Plan for Prevention of Blindness and Eye Care, aiming to persistently strengthen the government responsibilities, improve the tertiary blindness prevention and treatment network, strengthen the construction of personnel teams for prevention and treatment of blindness, and determinedly enhance the ability of eye care service at the primary level [1].

In recent years, the Chinese government has issued a series of policies for advancing the construction and development of medical complex, promoting the construction of the hierarchical medical system, and comprehensively improving the comprehensive diagnosis and treatment ability of county-level hospitals. The government has also developed comprehensive policies in the field of eye health [2], such as the policies encouraging ophthalmology department of tertiary hospitals, eye hospitals and ophthalmology department of county hospitals, primary health care institutes to cooperate vertically in improving eye disease diagnosis and treatment; strengthening and constructing communication and cooperation among ophthalmic institutions, disease control centers or eye disease prevention and treatment institutions, and low vision rehabilitation centers; taking the opportunity of reform of county public hospitals and counterpart aid from tertiary hospitals to hospitals in poor counties to give a big push to capacity building at the county level; incorporating primary eye care services into the primary health care system; strengthening the eye disease prevention and treatment at primary level, especially in rural areas, and exploring and establishing primary eye disease prevention and treatment models.

On December 6, 1984, the Chinese government established the National Committee for the Prevention of Blindness, consisting of professionals with experience in the prevention and treatment of blindness and the ability to provide professional guidance. As a professional organization for preventing blindness in China, its main duty is to, under the leadership of the National Health Commission of the People's Republic of China, develop blindness prevention and treatment plans, assist the National Health Commission of the People's Republic of China and health administrative departments at all levels in implementing the National Plan for the Prevention of Blindness, organize training for professionals, study and promote the appropriate ophthalmology techniques, and hold academic exchange activities regarding the prevention and treatment of blindness. The National Committee for the Prevention of Blindness, after its establishment, immediately started the national epidemiological survey on the prevention of blindness, the compilation of teaching materials for the training of blindness prevention workers at the county level, and the establishment of demonstration projects for blindness prevention in advanced counties. In addition, it also guided the establishment of provincial (autonomous regions and municipalities directly under the central government) and municipal committees for the prevention of blindness, as well as the eye disease prevention and treatment networks, namely national-provincial (autonomous region, municipality directly under the central government)-municipal level and county-township-village networks. The prevention and treatment networks have enabled China to smoothly conduct the eye health work, which has improved the coordination and implementation efficiency of eye health institutions, fully mobilized the enthusiasm, initiative and creativity of all levels, and gathered the force of eye care personnel and social sectors, thereby ensuring that the national blindness prevention policies can be timely implemented at the primary level, effectively improving and strengthening the awareness of the public on eye health, and popularizing the national eye health policies among the people.

China Disabled Persons' Federation (CDPF) has also made great efforts in providing eye health services. It has been engaging in the epidemiological survey, prevention, rehabilitation, as well as training of professional talents in the field of blindness and low vision, and organizing experts and academic bodies to hold International Low Vision Rehabilitation Forum and organize the training for low vision rehabilitation backbone talents.

II. Eye Health Plan

Over the years, the national health administrations have been developing the national blindness prevention and eye health plan, for guiding the work of blindness prevention in all provinces (autonomous regions and municipalities directly under the central government) in China. The "7th 5-Year National Plan for Prevention of Blindness and Eye Care (1988-

1990)" was the first blindness prevention and eye care plan, which stated the goal, major tasks, pilots, and supporting measures of blindness prevention, and also emphasized talent training, health care service capability, and development of eye disease prevention and treatment plan in schools. In addition, the primary eye health care plan involved the compilation of teaching materials, holding of training courses, training of primary health personnel, collection of data on blindness and low vision, health education, and establishment of an effective referral system. Meanwhile, the establishment of an information monitoring system and the improvement of the registration report and data collection system were emphasized in other related work, so as to gradually form a network. Moreover, the focus should be put on collecting information on blindness prevention in pilot areas, carrying out general treatment based on the unified national epidemiological basis, uniformly organizing ophthalmic medical teams of an appropriate scale to assist in the treatment of cataract in pilot areas, and combining professional institutions with primary eye care personnel to persistently increase the operation rate, thus ensuring that the number of treated blind people reaches 60% of the existing treatable blind people. The plan also specified the establishment and improvement of the research system, and qualified scientific research centers (institutes) in provinces should take the responsibility of solving urgent technical problems in blindness prevention, fully reflecting the characteristics of the times [3].

In 1992, the Chinese government issued the *Notice on National Plan of Blindness Prevention and Primary Eye Care in 1991-2000* (WYF [1992] No. 1), which was prepared based on the global strategic goal of "Health for All by the Year 2000" proposed by the World Health Organization (WHO). The work measures became more comprehensive than before, and the related plan and its requirements were proposed to strengthen the construction of committees for the prevention of blindness in provinces (autonomous regions and municipalities directly under the central government) and cities, establish blindness prevention teams, train professionals, incorporate primary eye care into primary health care, persistently develop and consolidate advanced counties for blindness prevention and treatment, prevent common eye diseases, reduce the number of new blind people, strengthen scientific research on the prevention and treatment of blindness, and standardize the primary eye care work [4].

In 2006, for further advancing the work of prevention and treatment of blindness, laying a solid foundation for the ultimate realization of the strategic goal of eliminating avoidable blindness by 2020, and protecting the health of the public, as well as promoting the coordinated development of the economy and society, the Chinese government issued the *National Plan for the Prevention of Blindness (2006-2010)*(WYF [2006] No. 282), which requires the strengthening of the leadership, the improvement of organizational structure, and the integration of social resources, the enhancement of the construction of the teams for blindness prevention and treatment, as well as the building of the ability of the teams for blindness prevention and treatment at the primary level. Moreover, it should also create the demonstration counties (districts) for prevention and treatment of blindness and cataract barrier-free counties (districts), strengthen medical and rehabilitation assistance for the poor visually impaired persons, organize publicity and education on prevention and treatment of blindness, and strengthen the corresponding investigation and research, so as to establish an information system for blindness prevention [5].

In 2012, the Ministry of Health and CDPF issued the *National Plan for the Prevention of Blindness (2012-2015)*(WYZF [2012] No. 52), in which, it was stated that there were a large number of patients with blindness and low vision in China due to the large population. In addition, insufficiency, uneven distribution, and low quality of ophthalmic medical resources, insufficient eye care service ability at the primary level, as well as incomplete information system, were mentioned. Therefore, the following suggestions were made: further establishing and improving the network for blindness prevention and treatment, strengthening the construction of the teams for blindness prevention and treatment, preventing leading blinding eye diseases, and carrying out low vision rehabilitation tasks, providing publicity and education on prevention and treatment of blindness, developing the guidelines for preventing common leading blinding eye diseases at the primary level, and further improving the information reporting system of cataract surgery [6].

In 2016, the National Health and Family Planning Commission issued *The 13ᵗʰ 5-Year National Eye Health Plan (2016-2020)*(GWYF [2016] No. 57). The title of the plan changed from National Plan for the Prevention of Blindness to National Eye Health Plan, indicating that the work of prevention and treatment of blindness in China has now entered a new level. As required in this plan, the governments at all levels should incorporate the prevention and treatment of eye diseases into the health development plan and poverty alleviation through health promotion work. Meanwhile, the government should also strengthen the communication and coordination with the CDPF, as well as other divisions in the fields of education, civil affairs, and finance. The measures in seven aspects were clarified in this plan, involving the improvement of the eye disease prevention and treatment service system; the strengthening of the construction of personnel teams, and the promotion of sustainable development; the prevention of major eye diseases that may cause blindness and visual impairment; the standardization of practice in the low vision rehabilitation; the conduct of publicity and education on eye health; the enhancement of data collection and information construction; and the improvement of the working mechanism of "leadership by government, cooperation among sectors" [1].

III. Changes in eye health policies

Since the 7ᵗʰ 5-Year National Plan, the Chinese government has been creating a positive policy environment for eye health. Under the high attention of the party and government, there was a change in the major blinding eye diseases, namely from infectious diseases (such as trachoma) to metabolic, chronic, and age-related eye diseases, under joint efforts of all sectors. Priority has been given to myopia in children and adolescents, high myopia-related fundus diseases, diabetic retinopathy, and age-related macular disease. National policies have been revised with the times, and the focus of blindness prevention has changed from the prevention and treatment of blindness to management of eye health and prevention of eye diseases [2]. The original blindness prevention and treatment plan has been updated to an eye health plan.

80% of the leading blinding eye diseases are preventable and controllable [7] require early detection and appropriate timely intervention. Therefore, the work pattern has changed from blindness prevention and treatment-focused pattern to multi-aspect eye health management. At present, more attention should be paid to primary eye care, which should be incorporated into primary health care. In addition, the management of ophthalmic diseases should be incorporated into the management of chronic diseases, and the eye health files should be kept, and long-term management mechanisms, such as eye health follow-up, should be established. With the changing of blindness prevention programs from the previous "blood transfusion" mode to the "hematopoiesis" mode, the focus of blindness prevention programs has changed from the provision of assistance and free treatment to training. In the past, the projects for blindness prevention were mainly conducted by medical teams dispatched, while in recent years, the projects such as "Standardized Training to Elevate Eyecare in Rural China" have been organized to cultivate professional talents, strengthen the local soft power, namely the mastery of technologies and service capacity of talents, and thus gradually creating a sustainable development model.

References

1. National Health and Family Planning Commission of the People's Republic of China. *Notice on release of the 13th 5-year national plan of eye health (2016-2020) by the national health and family planning commission* (GWYF [2016] No. 57)[EB/OL].(2016-11-09)[2020-04-12]. www. nhc. gov. cn/zwgk/zxgzjh/201611/9463 afb00ac84910bb3c22f8629cf90a. shtml.

2. National Health and Family Planning Commission of the People's Republic of China. *Notice on doing a better job in the construction of a hierarchical diagnosis and treatment system* (GWYF [2018] No. 28) [EB/OL].(2018-08-07)[2020-04-12]. http://www. nhc. gov. cn/xxgk/pages/viewdocument. jsp ? dispatchDate=&staticUrl=/yzygj/s3594q/201808/1c4adec50bfb4bf9b0803a5940b8bf14. shtml.

3. Ministry of Health of the People's Republic of China. *Notice on issuing the outline of the national plan*

for prevention of blindness and seventh 5-year plan for national blindness prevention and eye health [EB/OL].(1988-07-14)[2020-04-13]. http://www. moheyes. com/News/Details/9854fdd1-b63b-4254-b4f6-f51b2bc210ab.

4. Editorial Board of China Health Statistics Yearbook. *China health statistics yearbook (1993)* [M]. Beijng: People's Medical Publishing House, 1993: 181.

5. Ministry of Health of the People's Republic of China. *Notice on issuing the national plan for the prevention of blindness (2006-2010)*(WYF [2006] No. 282)[EB/OL].(2006-07-26)[2020-04-13]. http://www. nhc. gov. cn/wjw/gfxwj/201304/e6a33b8930ba445da6988ca012562d75. shtml.

6. Ministry of Health of the People's Republic of China, China Disabled Person's Federation. *Notice on issuing the national plan for the prevention of blindness (2012-2015)*(WYZF [2012] No. 52)[EB/OL](2012-07-27) [2020-04-13]. http://www. nhc. gov. cn/jnr/qgayrbmgz/201406/29f041a9126c484e87b8e7c36dc91b24. shtml.

7. World Health Organization. *Universal eye health: a global action plan 2014-2019*.[EB/OL].(2013-05-24) [2020-04-19]. https://apps. who. int/iris/bitstream/handle/10665/105937/9789245506560_chi. pdf; jsessionid= 938CF4336F6ED37306821D82CE8076BB？ sequence=9.

Chapter II   Eye Disease Prevention and Treatment Work Pattern with Chinese Characteristics

Blindness prevention in China has been adhering to the pattern of "leadership by government, multi-sectoral collaboration, and social participation", aiming at providing overall, equal and accessible eye care services for the public.

I. Government coordination and policy guidance

The construction of Healthy China is an important foundation for building a moderately well-off society in an all-around way and basically realizing socialist modernization. It is also a national strategy to comprehensively improve the health of the Chinese people and realize the harmonious development between people's health and economy and society. Moreover, it is also a major initiative to actively participate in global health governance and fulfill the commitment of the "2030 Agenda for Sustainable Development"[1]. Eye health, as an important part of national health, should be persistently promoted, so as to further improve the eye health of the public[2].

By the end of 2019, basic medical insurance had covered 1,354,360,000 people, with a coverage rate of over 95%, basically achieving full coverage[3]. In 2020, cataract was included in the scope of diseases of Special Fund for Poor Rural Population with Major Diseases[4]. In addition, in order to further improve the affordability of medical care and achieve equalization of public medical care, the government adopted several specific medical reform measures, such as day surgery, reduction of the length of stay and waiting time, lowering of medical expenses, and effective use of the beds[5]. The implementation of the medicine zero markups policy in public hospitals has brought real benefits to the patients, and prevented the phenomenon of "returning to poverty because of illness" [6].

In 2016, the National Health and Family Planning Commission issued *The 13th 5-Year National Eye Health Plan (2016-2020)*(GWYF [2016] No. 57), in which, the responsibilities, tasks and requirements of eye hospitals at all levels were clarified, including ophthalmology departments of general hospitals, maternity and child care institution and primary medical and health institutions with ophthalmology departments. All these hospitals and institutions were asked to provide the comprehensive, equal, and accessible ophthalmic medical services. The professionals from all national and provincial committees for the prevention of blindness, as well as the societies and associations of ophthalmology, should exert their strength and organize the training for primary ophthalmic personnel and related health workers, to improve their capacity in diagnosis and treatment of common eye diseases and enable them to play the role in guiding the provision of primary ophthalmic medical services, thus further implementing hierarchical diagnosis and treatment [2]. In view of the large difference between resources in urban and rural areas, county-level hospitals (principal implementers of primary blindness prevention and treatment work) still suffered from weakness in eye health work and lack of talents. On May 18, 2016, the National Committee for the Prevention of Blindness launched "Standardized Training to Elevate Eyecare in Rural China", aiming to train the teams for providing high-quality ophthalmic services in county-level hospitals. In addition, based on the model of "tertiary training", the project also aimed to establish a standardized training model for the primary eye care service capacity building in China. By the end of 2019, the project had completed the training in more than 70 county-level hospitals, involving about 350 members of county-level ophthalmology teams, 3,070 country doctors and 1,686 trainers. Furthermore, it had also screened 487,308 adults for cataract, and 328,317 children for refractive error.

II. Technical support from academic bodies

Myopia in children and adolescents has become a common concern in society. In August 2018, Xi Jinping, general secretary of the Communist Party of China Central Committee, proposed and emphasized that "the whole society must take actions to jointly take good care of children's eyes and enable them to have a bright future". In order to further advance the prevention and treatment of myopia, eight ministries, including the Ministry of Education and National Health Commission, jointly issued the *Implementation Plan for Comprehensive Prevention and Control of Myopia in Children and Adolescents* (JTY [2018] No. 3) [7]. For implementing Xi's instructions, organizing the work in a better manner, and giving full play to the guiding role of the National Committee for the Prevention of Blindness, ophthalmologists, and ophthalmic institutions in eye health, the National Committee for the Prevention of Blindness set up an expert group on myopia prevention and control, aiming to provide professional and technical advice on prevention and treatment of myopia for the government and health departments at all levels, provide guidance for medical institutions and eye care personnel to scientifically correct myopia, and assist in the epidemiological survey related to the prevention and treatment of myopia. In addition, the National Committee for the Prevention of Blindness, as entrusted by the National Health Commission, organized experts to compile the *Guidelines for Myopia Prevention*, *Guidelines for Strabismus Prevention*, and *Guidelines for Amblyopia Prevention* [8].

China has the largest population with type 2 diabetes in the world. With the increase in the number of diabetic patients, the prevalence and blindness rate of diabetic retinopathy have been increasing year by year. Diabetic retinopathy has become the leading blinding disease in the working-age population. Evidence-based medicine studies showed that the risk of diabetic retinopathy in diabetic patients could be significantly reduced through the strict control of blood glucose, blood lipid, and blood pressure, as well as the regular fundus screening. The intervention measures for patients with early diabetic retinopathy could significantly reduce the blinding rate. At present, 87% of diabetic patients accept treatment in medical institutions at the county level or below, but the basic diagnosis and treatment measures and appropriate technologies for diabetic retinopathy are mainly available in tertiary medical institutions [9]. Therefore, the National Committee for the Prevention of Blindness organized experts to compile the *Guidelines for the Prevention and Treatment of Diabetic Retinopathy* (*Primary Edition*) and the *Guideline for Hierarchical Diagnosis and Treatment of Diabetic Retinopathy* [9, 10], which, on the basis of a hierarchical medical system, could further improve the standardized treatment at the primary level, establish an effective model of early screening, diagnosis, referral, and treatment, and also reduce the disease burden [10].

On September 9, 2017, the National Committee for the Prevention of Blindness organized 146 hospitals to formally establish the National Ophthalmology Alliance, aiming to concentrate the professional force of the national ophthalmic community, and make full use of cutting-edge technologies, to share various resources, including experts, clinics, scientific research, teaching, and patients, and also implement the patient-oriented hierarchical diagnosis, treatment and referral system. Meanwhile, the National Ophthalmology Alliance also intended to improve the overall quality of national ophthalmology talents through strengthening the standardized training for ophthalmologists and eye care talents. In addition, it also established a scientific research platform for promoting the development of clinical scientific research and transformation of results, guiding the research direction, improving research level, and realizing the sharing of multi-center clinical data and case resources among member units, as well as systematically understanding the current situation of eye health based on big data analysis, thereby providing a basis for the development of blindness prevention and treatment policies. The "Chinese Glaucoma Study Alliance" was formally established in 2014, aiming to further conduct research on glaucoma genetics and construct a scientific research platform for high-quality multi-center clinical research, train clinical researchers and improve their clinical research capabilities, thus promoting new technologies and new projects. For further promoting the diagnosis and treatment of glaucoma in hospitals at all levels, and effectively implementing the guidelines and specifications for diagnosis and treatment of glaucoma, the Alliance established an Electric Data Capture (EDC) system for realizing effective quality control of the data. In the annual national meeting, the Chinese Ophthalmological Society set up the keynote report on blindness prevention at the plenary session, and held the session for blindness prevention, to discuss new concepts, new developments, new technologies and new ideas of blindness prevention. In view of the common leading blinding eye diseases in China, various professional groups of Chinese Ophthalmological Society have successively launched several expert consensus or guidelines: *Expert Consensus on Diagnosis and Treatment of Primary Glaucoma in China* launched by the Glaucoma Committee; *Guidelines for Clinical Diagnosis and Treatment of Diabetic Retinopathy* launched by the Retinopathy Committee; *Expert Consensus on Clinical Diagnosis and Treatment of Infectious Keratopathy* launched by the Keratopathy Committee; *Expert Consensus on Prevention and Control of High Myopia* launched by the Ophthalmology & Optometry Committee; *Expert Consensus on the Treatment of Acute Bacterial Endophthalmitis after Cataract Surgery in China* launched by the Cataract Committee; and *Expert Consensus on Diagnosis of Amblyopia* launched by the Strabismus and Pediatric Ophthalmology Committee, based on which, the diagnosis and treatment of leading blinding eye diseases have been standardized, thus contributing to the reduction of the blinding rate of leading blinding eye diseases in China.

Since the founding of the People's Republic of China, the guidelines for health work have been revised three times, and no modification has been made to the principle "prevention first". Most eye diseases are chronic diseases, of which, 80% can be prevented and controlled [11], and the overcrowding in large hospitals can only be alleviated through paying attention to the prevention and control of eye diseases. During the "13th 5-Year Plan" Period, the key emphasis in eye health was turned to "eye health services" from "prevention and treatment of blindness". Eye health required emphasizing the intervention based on the influencing factors of eye health, and adhering to the principle of "prevention first and primary care-centered" [2]. Society of Public Health Ophthalmology, Chinese Preventive Medicine Association, as the first professional organization formally established for combining public health with prevention of eye diseases, aims to promote the development of public health ophthalmology, improve the level of ophthalmology public health and preventive medicine, and effectively improve the ability to prevent and control eye diseases in China. The Society has strengthened the combination of ophthalmology with public health. It holds training courses for doctors at primary level institutions each year, aiming to enable them to have the mindset and awareness of public health ophthalmology. In addition, it also irregularly holds high-level academic conferences and forums focusing on hot spots and focal points regarding public health ophthalmology. During the epidemic of COVID-19, its council members proposed suggestions on ophthalmic protection from the perspectives of preventive medicine and ophthalmology, and also provided comprehensive, meticulous and practical suggestions on protective actions based on the guidance of the government. They also published the *Suggestions from Ophthalmic Experts on Eye Protection During the Corona Virus Disease 2019 Epidemic* (Chinese and English versions) and the *Eye Protection Manual During the Epidemic of COVID-19*, making its own contribution to the joint fight against COVID-19.

III. Active participation of private hospitals and social organizations

At present, public hospitals are still the main providers of ophthalmic medical services, however, in recent years, social capital has entered into the field of health care by virtue of a series of medical reform policies promoting private hospitals, and private hospitals have become an important part of medical resources in China. The private eye hospitals could make up for the relative insufficiency of ophthalmic resources, and introduce advanced management models and service systems by virtue of the flexibility of high-quality private eye hospitals. At the end of 2018, the number of ophthalmic beds in medical and health institutions reached 130,000 in China, and the number of annual outpatients reached 120 million [12]. The related report showed that the market size of private eye institutions accounted for one-fifth of the national eye service market. In addition, with the improvement of living standards, the demand for middle and high-end ophthalmic services has been increasing day by day, such as eye health management and special eye services, leading to multi-level and diversified demand for ophthalmic medical services. The development of private eye hospitals could improve the overall utilization efficiency of ophthalmic medical service resources, and meet the requirements of urban and rural residents for multi-level ophthalmic medical services.

With the development of eye health in China, many non-governmental organizations (NGOs) have actively participated in blindness prevention in China. In 1997, national health administrations and Lions Clubs International jointly launched the "Sight First-China Action". Since then, three phases of work have been completed. In Phase I and Phase II, a total of 548 medical teams were dispatched, who completed 5.03 million cataract operations, helped to construct 210 county-level hospitals, established 6 regional training centers and 25 provincial-level training bases, and also trained more than 60,000 eye health personnel. In Phase III, the project "Elimination of Blinding Trachoma by 2016 in China" was launched for evaluation, screening, and treatment of trachoma [13].

Lifeline Express, established in 1997, had provided services in 187 service sites in 121 regions of 28 provinces (autonomous regions and municipalities directly under the central government), and implemented sight restoration surgeries for more than 210,000 poor cataract patients by the end of 2019. "Diabetic Retinopathy Screening" project had established 40 centers for diabetic retinopathy screening in 21 provinces (autonomous regions and municipalitiesdirectly under the central government), helped 235 doctors to obtain the internationally certified qualification of diabetic retinopathy image reading, and screened a total of more than 190,000 diabetic patients, including 6,700 diabetic patients on the verge of blindness.

Orbis International has engaged in blindness prevention activities in China since 1982. So far, it has completed 41 flying eye hospital projects in China, and completed 230 projects in 32 provinces, municipalities and autonomous regions. Moreover, it has trained 70,000 health workers and helped more than 17 million people.

The Fred Hollows Foundation started eliminating avoidable blindness in China in 1998. Up to now, it has trained more than 30,000 health workers, performed vision screening for nearly 3 million people, and treated more than 1.4 million patients with eye diseases.

"Project Vision", initiated in Hong Kong in 2004, was designated to develop a mode of sustainable blindness prevention in China. As of October 2018, it had established 30 poverty alleviation eye centers in 10 provincial administrative regions completed 163,839 cataract operations, and trained more than 140 cataract surgeons in China.

The Asian Foundation for the Prevention of Blindness has committed to blindness prevention and treatment in developing countries in Asia. It established "China Mobile Eye Treatment Center Project" in 1995, which had helped more than 640,000 poor cataract patients to recover vision by 2019.

References

1. State Council of the People's Republic of China. *Healthy China 2030 planning outline*.[EB/OL].(2016-10-25) [2020-04-05]. http://www. gov. cn/xinwen/2016-10/25/content_5124174. htm.
2. National Health and Family Planning Commission of the People's Republic of China. *Notice on release of the 13th 5-year national plan of eye health (2016-2020) by the National Health and Family Planning Commission* (GWYH [2016] No. 57)[EB/OL].(2016-11-09)[2020-04-05]. www. nhc. gov. cn/zwgk/zxgzjh/ 201611/9463afb00ac84910bb3c22f8629cf90a. shtml.
3. National Healthcare Security Administration of the People's Republic of China. *Health care development bulletin 2019*.[EB/OL].(2020-03-30)[2020-04-05]. http://www. nhsa. gov. cn/art/2020/3/30/art_7_2930. html.

4. National Health Commission of the People's Republic of China. *Notice on further expanding the scope of special treatment diseases for rural poor population.*(GWBYH [2020] No. 338)[EB/OL]. http://www. xinhuanet. com/2019-05/14/c_1124491553. htm. 2020-04-05.

5. SHI LIQUN, XIA ZHONGDANG, PAN YUNLONG. Promotion of the management of day surgery standardization [J]. Modern hospital, 2015, 15 (11): 9-10.

6. XU JUNHUA. Effect and measures of drugs zero-profit in the public hospitals [J]. Modern economic information. 2014,(10): 316-325.

7. Ministry of Education of the People's Republic of China. *Notice of eight departments including the Ministry of Education on issuing the implementation plan for comprehensive prevention and control of myopia among children and adolescents* (JTY [2018] No. 3).[EB/OL].(2018-04-05)[2020-08-30]. http://www. moe. gov. cn/srcsite/A17/moe_943/s3285/201808/t20180830_346672. html.

8. National Health Commission of the People's Republic of China. *Notice on issuing the guidelines for myopia prevention, guidelines for strabismus prevention and guidelines for amblyopia prevention.* (GWBYH [2018] No. 393)[EB/OL].(2018-06-01)[2020-04-05]. http://www. moe. gov. cn/jyb_xwfb/xw_zt/moe_357/jyzt_2019n/2019_zt7/zcjj/bw/201904/t20190428_379876. html.

9. National Health and Family Planning Commission of the People's Republic of China. *Notice of the general office of national health commission on issuing the guideline for hierarchical diagnosis and treatment of diabetic retinopathy.*(GWBYH [2017] No. 280)[EB/OL].(2017-04-01)[2020-04-05]. http://www. nhc. gov. cn/yzygj/s7653/201704/3524f29f1599419aa04bbe4e068c962a. shtml.

10. National Committee for the Prevention of Blindness. *Guidelines for the prevention and treatment of diabetic retinopathy (primary edition)*[M]. Beijng: People's Medical Publishing House, 2017: 2.

11. World Health Organization. *Universal eye health: a global action plan 2014-2019.*[EB/OL].(2013-05-24)[2020-04-19]. https://apps. who. int/iris/bitstream/handle/10665/105937/9789245506560_chi. pdf; jsessionid=938CF4336F6ED37306821D82CE8076BB ? sequence=9.

12. National Health Commission of the People's Republic of China. *China health statistics yearbook.* [M]. Beijng: Peking Union Medical College Press, 2020.

13. WANG NINGLI, HU AILIAN, HUGH R TAYLOr. *Trachoma* [M]. Beijng: People's Medical Publishing House, 2015: 39.

Chapter III   Progress under "VISION 2020" Initiative

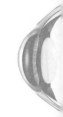

I. "VISION 2020" initiative

"VISION 2020", a global initiative initiated by the WHO and the International Agency for the Prevention of Blindness (IAPB) on February 18, 1999, aims to eliminate avoidable blindness around the world by 2020 and reverse the trend that avoidable visual impairment may double between 1990 and 2020. It also intends to improve the awareness of key population with respect to main causes and solutions of avoidable blindness; develop and guarantee the resources necessary for the prevention and treatment of blindness; and promote the planning, development and implementation of national projects in various countries around the world under "VISION 2020". Three core strategies, namely disease control in combination with primary health care, development of human resources, and infrastructure construction and application of appropriate technologies, are applied under this initiative [1-2].

In 2006, the World Health Assembly (WHA) passed the resolution WHA59.25, which added the prevention of avoidable visual impairment in the "VISION 2020" initiative on the basis of the resolution WHA56.26 on the prevention of avoidable blindness adopted in 2003. At WHA 2013, Resolution 66.4 "Universal eye health: A global action plan 2014—2019" was passed, which was still a part of "VISION 2020", but its goal was adjusted to "reduce the prevalence of avoidable visual impairment by 25% by 2019"(compared with the baseline prevalence in 2010). Compared with the original goal of eliminating avoidable visual impairment by 2020, this goal is more achievable [3]. The ultimate goal of this resolution is to reduce avoidable visual impairment that may become a public health issue, and make all people with unavoidable visual impairment enjoy rehabilitation services [4].

II. "VISION 2020" in China

In September 1999, "VISION 2020" was officially launched in the Western Pacific Region. China was the first country to launch "VISION 2020". Wenkang Zhang, Minister of the Ministry of Health, signed the Declaration in Beijing, and solemnly made a commitment to the elimination of avoidable blindness by 2020. Major cause of avoidable blindness includes cataract, trachoma, onchocerciasis, childhood blindness, low vision and refractive error, of which, onchocerciasis does not exist in China, but only in a few countries in Africa and Latin America [4]. In 2006, the Chinese government launched the *National Plan for the Prevention of Blindness* (*2006-2010*) (WYF [2006] No. 282). By the end of 2008, 27 provinces, municipalities, and autonomous regions had developed their own 5-year plans or drafts for prevention and treatment of blindness [5]. In 2012, the Chinese government launched the *National Plan for the Prevention of Blindness* (*2012-2015*)(WYZF [2012] No. 52) referring to the core strategy of "VISION 2020" based on the work progress achieved during the "11th 5-Year Plan" Period. In 2016, according to the overall requirements for the construction of Healthy China and deepening the reform of the medical and health system, as well as the WHO's resolution "Universal Eye Health: A Global Action Plan 2014-2019", *The 13th 5-Year National Eye Health Plan* (*2016-2020*)(GWYF [2016] No. 57) was issued, aiming to persistently promote the public eye health during the "13th 5-Year Plan" period.

While implementing this action, China integrated the prevention and treatment of avoidable visual impairment into the national health plan and provision of health services and integrated ophthalmic medical services into the medical service system, so as to persistently improve the blindness prevention and treatment network in rural areas. Furthermore, China also held the survey on ophthalmic medical resources and epidemiology of eye diseases and strengthened publicity and education on the prevention and treatment of blindness. The prevention and treatment of blindness should not only focus on eye diseases [6-7]. In addition, the pattern "led by government, participated by all parties" has been established through establishing and improving national, provincial and municipal blindness prevention and treatment management systems, technical guidance systems and service systems and fully mobilizing the blindness prevention resources [8]. In order to increase the awareness of the major causes of and solutions to avoidable blindness in key populations, June 6 was set as National Eye Care Day themed prevention and treatment of avoidable blindness [9]. Remarkable progress has been achieved in the development of human resources and construction of infrastructure. The quantity of county-level hospitals that can provide ophthalmic medical services and those with independent ophthalmology departments increased from 1,995 and 1,033 in 2003 [10] to 3,478 and 1,807 in 2018, and the number of ophthalmologists increased from 19,100 in 2003 [10] to 44,800 in 2018. As for the promotion of suitable techniques, several plans and guidelines have been issued: the *Technical Specifi-cations for Eye and Vision Care for Children*, *Guidelines for Suitable Techniques for Preven-tion and Treatment of Myopia in Children and Adolescents*, and *Guidelines for the Treatment of Preterm Infants with Oxygen and the Prevention and Treatment of Retinopathy*. The suit-able techniques for prevention and treatment of eye diseases have been promoted through the eye disease prevention and treatment network, which can improve the services for prevention and treatment of eye diseases, especially the ability of primary and rural areas to prevent and treat eye diseases.

Ⅲ. Progress in eliminating avoidable blindness

The avoidable blindness to be eliminated under "VISION 2020" involves cataract, trachoma, onchocerciasis, childhood blindness, low vision and refractive error, and we have no oncho-cerciasis in China.

Cataract is the leading blinding eye disease in China. Cataract surgery rate (CSR) is one of the three monitoring indicators in *Universal Eye Health*: *A Global Action Plan 2014-2019* launched by the WHO [11]. After making long-term efforts, including carrying out free treatment for cataract programs, gradually expanding the coverage of medical insurance, and improving ophthalmic service capacity of county-level medical institutions, CSR in China increased from 318 in 1999 [12] to 2,205 in 2017, realizing the goal proposed in *The 13th 5-Year National Eye Health Plan* in advance, namely increasing CSR to over 2,000 at the end of 2020(Fig.3-1).

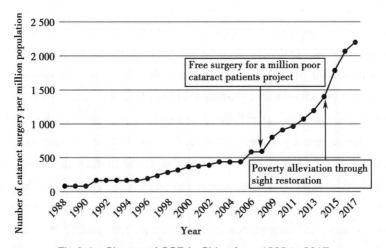

Fig.3-1   Change of CSR in China from 1998 to 2017

Trachoma, in addition to cataract, is also an eye disease concerned under the "VISION 2020" initiative. From the 1940s to the 1950s, trachoma was the leading blinding eye disease in

China. In 1987, the disability rate of trachoma accounted for 14.25% of all visual disabilities, and became the third leading cause. In 2006, the disability rate of trachoma decreased to 1.87%, which indicated that trachoma was no longer a major blinding eye disease in China. The evaluation conducted at the end of 2014 showed that the rate of active trachoma was less than 5% in children aged 1 to 9, and the rate of trachoma trichiasis was less than 0.1% in adults, achieving the goal of eliminating blinding trachoma proposed by the WHO [13]. At the World Health Assembly held in Switzerland in 2015, Bin Li, Director of the National Health and Family Planning Commission, officially announced that China met WHO's requirement for eliminating blinding trachoma in 2014, indicating that China reached the goal of eliminating blinding trachoma in advance. In 2019, the WHO certified the elimination of blinding trachoma in China based on the new procedures and standards.

Childhood blindness accounts for a relatively low proportion of all blindness, but considering the early onset age, disability adjusted life year and long time spent with disability, it would lead to a huge burden to the family and society. Studies have shown that childhood blindness in 1/3 to 1/2 children could be avoided or treated [14]. Eye diseases that can cause visual dysplasia and even low vision or blindness in children include retinopathy of prematurity, congenital cataract, congenital glaucoma, neonatal gonococcal conjunctivitis, amblyopia, strabismus, high refractive error, anisometropia, congenital ptosis, and retinoblastoma. Over the years, the Chinese government has been actively promoting early screening and treatment of childhood blindness, based on which, the incidence of retinopathy of prematurity decreased from 20.3% in 1990s to 10.8% in 2005 in Beijing, thus significantly lowering the blindness rate [15]. Since the issuance of the *Guidelines for the Treatment of Preterm Infants with Oxygen and the Prevention and Treatment of Retinopathy* [16] in 2004, the screening system led by one ophthalmology center and supported by multiple neonatal intensive care units has been basically formed in Beijing, Shanghai, Guangzhou, and Shenzhen, etc.

The Second China National Sample Survey on Disability in 2006 showed that in 51,328 children aged 0 to 6,193 had visual disability, with the visual disability rate of 3.76‰; 93 had genetic, congenital abnormalities or developmental disabilities, with the visual disability rate of 1.8‰; 61 had visual disability due to amblyopia, with the visual disability rate of 1.18‰; and 19 had refractive error, with the visual disability rate of 0.37‰. In 2013, in order to improve the quality of health care and further standardize the contents, methods, procedures and assessments of health care for children in all related fields, the *Notice on Issuing Technical Specifications for Children's Eye and Vision Care* (WBFSF [2013] No. 26) was issued. In 2019, the *Notice on Eye Care and Vision Inspection for Children Aged 0 to 6* (GWBFYF [2019] No. 9) was issued, which asked all institutions to accelerate the establishment and improvement of the Resident Electronic

Health Record Information System, realize electronic management of vision health records for children aged 0-6, and ensure that the contents of vision health records of the children aged 0 to 6 are complete, accurate, and extractable upon admission to schools. Such records should be timely transferred to the educational institutions. In addition, the statistical indicators of " The number of children aged 0 to 6 for eye care and vision inspection","The number of children aged 6 for vision inspection" and "The number of children aged 6 detected with poor vision"were added in the *Annual Report on Care and Health of Children Under Seven*. Every year, the medical and health institutions responsible for providing basic public health services should document records on eye care and vision inspection for children aged 0 to 6. In addition, the coverage of eye care and vision inspection and electronic vision health records of children aged 0-6 should also be incorporated into the assessment system. It is required that the annual coverage of eye care and vision inspection in children aged 0 to 6 should be more than 90% from 2019.

In 1991, low vision rehabilitation was incorporated in the *Outline on China's Disability Work in the 8th 5-year Plan Period* (1991—1995). The CDPF took low vision rehabilitation as one of its major tasks, and provided typoscopes for hundreds of thousands of low vision patients through setting up low vision rehabilitation departments, training personnel, developing and supplying visual aid devices, and publicizing the related knowledge. Based on the monograph *Clinical Low Vision* and national higher education textbook *Low Vision*, as well as training courses at all levels, a large number of low vision rehabilitation professionals and parents of children with low vision were trained. *The 13th 5-Year National Eye Health Plan* (*2016-2020*) (GWYF [2016] No. 57) clearly indicated that ophthalmology departments of tertiary general hospitals and eye hospitals should provide low-vision outpatient services. The hospitals with conditions should provide low vision rehabilitation services, and establish the cooperation and referral mechanism between ophthalmic institutions and low vision rehabilitation centers. In addition, they should also strengthen the team construction of talents in the field of low-vision, and promote sustainable development [9]. At the same time, the Ministry of Finance should increase investment to support the professional fitting of typoscopes and training for rehabilitation and strongly support the research and development of typoscopes with independent property rights.

Myopia, a type of refractive error, is an eye health problem with the highest incidence and the greatest span of age in the world. Retinopathy due to high myopia accounts for a high proportion of the causes of blindness. The prevention and treatment of uncorrected refractive error have become an important part of eye health work and been upgraded to a national strategy in China. Eight ministries and commissions jointly developed the *Implementation Plan for Comprehensive Prevention and Treatment of Myopia in Children and Adolescents* (JTY [2018]

No. 3) and issued a series of technical guides and prevention manuals. Local governments have successively launched the baseline survey on myopia rate in children and adolescents, organized experts for inspection on myopia survey and carried out a series of publicity activities named "prevention of myopia in children and adolescents" throughout China.

Under "VISION 2020", significant progress has been made in the prevention and treatment of blindness in China. Governments at all levels have attached great importance to and played a leading role in the prevention of blindness [17]. The prevention and treatment service system in ophthalmology departments of county-level hospitals is being gradually improved, and both quantity and service quality of county-level ophthalmological institutions are persistently increased and strengthened. Eye care teams are further built, and the quantity and quality of human resources are optimized. Great achievements have been made in the prevention and treatment of the leading blinding eye diseases, such as cataract and trachoma. The ophthalmic institutions are also better equipped. With that, eye health work has enjoyed rapid progress.

References

1. World Health Organization. What is VISION 2020？ [EB/OL].[2020-04-19]. https://www. who. int/blindness/ partnerships/vision2020/en/.

2. The International Agency for the Prevention of Blindness. VISION 2020 action plan 2006-2011.[EB/OL]. [2020-04-19]. https://www. iapb. org/resources/vision-2020-action-plan-2006-2011/.

3. The International Agency for the Prevention of Blindness. What is VISION 2020？ [EB/OL].[2020-04-19]. https://www. iapb. org/global-initiatives/vision-2020/what-is-vision-2020/.

4. HE SZ. Challenges of cataract restoration in the 21st century [J]. Chinese journal of ophthalmology, 2001, 037 (005): 321-324.

5. China National Blindness Prevention and Treatment. Introduction of "VISION 2020 "[EB/OL].(2013-01-01) [2020-04-17]. http://moheyes. com/News/Details/a8e735ab-32a9-4a38-a060-b269b9f24215.

6. ZHAO JL. To promote universal eye health to push forward sustaining development of the prevention of blindness in China [J]. Chinese journal of ophthalmology, 2014, 050 (003): 161-163.

7. HU X, ZHANG R, XU X, et al. Work together to make a new progress in China's blindness prevention and treatment [J]. National medical journal of China, 2013, 093 (047): 3731-3732.

8. National Health and Family Planning Commission of the People's Republic of China. *Notice of national health commission on issuing the 13th 5-year national eye health plan (2016-2020)*(GWYF [2016] No. 57)[EB/ OL].(2016-11-09)[2020-04-19]. http://www. nhc. gov. cn/wjw/ghjh/201611/9463afb00ac84910bb3c22f8629c f90a. shtml.

9. ANG XH, HU AL, WANG NL. From the prevention and treatment of blindness to the universal eye health [J]. Ophthalmology in China, 2017 (1): 9-11.

10. WANG YU. Statistical analysis report on the status of ophthalmology in China (2003)[Z]. 2004.

11. World Health Organization. Universal eye health: a global action plan 2014-2019.[EB/OL].(2013-05-24) [2020-04-19]. https://apps. who. int/iris/bitstream/handle/10665/105937/9789245506560_chi. pdf; jsessionid= 938CF4336F6ED37306821D82CE8076BB？ sequence=9.

12. GUAN HJ. Present status and development of prevention of blindness and ophthalmic epidemiologic studies in China [J]. Chinese journal of ophthalmology, 2010, 046 (010): 938-943.

13. WANG NL, HU AL. Enlightenment and thinking of blinding trachoma elimination in China [J]. Chinese journal of ophthalmology, 2015 (7): 484-486.

14. GOGATE P, MUHIT M, SHI LEI. Blindness and cataract in children in developing countries [J]. Journal of practical preventing blind, 2010, 005 (003): 93-95.

15. CHEN Y, FENG J, LI F, et al. Analysis of changes in characteristics of severe retinopathy of prematurity patients after screening guidelines were issued in China [J]. Retina. 2015, 35 (8): 1674-1679.

16. Ministry of Health of the People's Republic of China. *Notice of Ministry of Health on issuing the guidelines for the treatment of preterm infants with oxygen and the prevention and treatment of retinopathy* (WYF [2004] No. 104)[EB/OL].(2004-06-28)[2020-04-19]. http://www. nhc. gov. cn/bgt/pw10405/200 406/21c22c38dc004863bb5af817fb7753d0. shtml.

17. ZHAO JL. Chinese ophthalmologists should unswervingly promote "VISION 2020" [J]. Practical journal of clinical medicine, 2011, 7 (6): 1-3.

Chapter IV   Ophthalmic Resources

Ophthalmic resources are the key to ensuring people's access to eye health services, and the improvement of accessibility of ophthalmic resources is an important task for the implementation of the work of prevention and treatment of blindness. Over the past 20 years, China's eye health work has developed rapidly, with significant progress in ophthalmic resources construction. The service system for the prevention and treatment of ocular diseases in county-level hospitals has been strengthened, with the quantity and quality of human resources persistently optimized and ophthalmic devices and equipment better equipped.

I. Increase of the number of county-level ophthalmology institutions, and strengthening of service capabilities

An important action for China to improve the overall ability of medical services and lead the development of county-level hospitals is to enhance the comprehensive ability of county-level hospitals. For realizing the general goal of "VISION 2020", the key is to construct ophthalmology in county-level medical institutions. Under the continuous promotion of various policies and blindness prevention projects, county-level medical institutions have significantly improved their eye health service capabilities with learning opportunities provided by various eye health related projects. Moreover, the eye health professionals were encouraged and supported to participate in professional training and continued studies and to improve their services capacities by carrying out eye disease screening activities. In 2003, the number of county-level hospitals with the ability to provide ophthalmic medical services and those with independent ophthalmology departments reached 1,995 and 1,033, respectively [1], and then 3,359 and 1,463 [2,3] in 2014. Under the promotion of various blindness prevention policies, ophthalmic institutions in county-level hospitals have vigorously developed. National survey on ophthalmic resources in 2018 showed that the number of county-level hospitals with the ability to provide ophthalmic medical services and those with independent ophthalmology departments was 3,478 and 1,807, respectively. More than 10% of county-level hospitals established independent ophthalmology departments between 2014 and 2018. Primary ophthalmic teams have become more professional and are able to provide better medical services, constituting a qualified platform for primary blindness prevention activities in China. With the increase in the quantity of ophthalmic institutions and enhancement of their service quality, the total number of outpatients of county-level hospitals increased from 9.41 million visits in 2003 to 31.4 million visits in 2014 [1,2]. The number of outpatients in county-level hospitals reached 64.19 million visits in 2018, 2 times of that in 2014, as shown in Fig.4-1, ensuring convenient primary ophthalmic services for more patients.

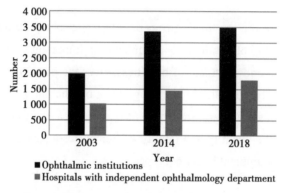

Fig.4-1   Ophthalmic institutions in county-level
hospitals in 2003,2014 and 2018

II. Growing of ophthalmic personnel team

From the "10th 5-Year Plan" to the "13th 5-Year Plan", the teams of ophthalmologists in China have been growing under the promotion of blindness prevention policies and projects. They laid a solid foundation of human resources needed for the promotion of the prevention and treatment of blindness. The survey indicated that the number of ophthalmologists increased from 19,100 in 2003 to 28,300 in 2006, and then 36,300 in 2014 [1,3]. The survey on national ophthalmic resources in 2018 showed that the number of ophthalmologists had reached 44,800 (Fig.4-2). In addition, the number of ophthalmologists in county-level hospitals also increased greatly, from 8,769 in 1998 to 9,965 in 2003, 13,200 in 2014 [1,3,4], and then 14, 200 in 2018 (Fig.4-3). The proportion of intermediate and senior doctors increased from 45.35% in 1998 to 59.73% in 2014, forming a more reasonably structured staff composition [3,4]. The Chinese government has long been making efforts in the prevention of blindness caused by cataracts. Since the 1980s, the government has clarified the goals of and actions for the prevention of blindness caused by cataracts at different stages in various blindness prevention plans and policies, and also vigorously strengthened the construction of ophthalmology in county-level general hospitals. As a result, the cataract surgery ability of county-level hospitals has been greatly improved. In 2018, the number of doctors capable of performing cataract surgery was 13,835,2.33 times of that in 2000 (5,939) [5] (Fig.4-4). At present, the total number of ophthalmologists in China is 44,800, namely 1.6 ophthalmologists per 50,000 people [6], exceeding WHO's requirement of "one ophthalmologist per 50,000 people" in Asia [7].

Nursing staff plays a major and important role in eye care services, and the number and composition of nursing staff could not only determine the quality of ophthalmic nursing but also directly affect the quality and safety of medical services. Since China made the commitment to "VISION 2020" in 1999, the number of ophthalmic nurses has been significantly increased under the promotion of various policies, from 16,100 in 2003 to 22,400 in 2006, and then 44,100 in 2014 [1,8] (Fig.4-2). Furthermore, in county-level hospitals, the number of ophthalmic nurses increased from 7,886 in 1998 to 7,978 in 2003, and then 15,400 in 2014 [1,2,4] (Fig.4-3). Meanwhile, the ophthalmologists-nurses ratio gradually became optimal, from 1 : 1.21 in 2014 to 1 : 0.79 in 2006, increasing by 53.16% in 8 years [2].

Uncorrected refractive error is one of the main causes of visual impairment around the world, accounting for about 42% [9]. In 2018, the overall prevalence of myopia in children and adolescents was 53.6%, with a prevalence of 14.5% in children aged 6, 36.0% in elementary school students, 71.6% in junior high school students, and 81.0% in senior high school students [10]. The prevalence of myopia in Chinese students is growing higher and with a younger onset age. With support from national policies for blindness prevention, the number of optometrists increased from 1,487 in 2006 to 3,950 in 2014, with an increase of 1.5 times [3] (Fig.4-5), and from 3,950 in 2014 to 6,418 in 2018, with an increase of nearly 1 time. However, compared with the huge myopic population in China, there are still no sufficient qualified full-time optometrists, indicating there is a long way to go regarding the training of professional optometrists.

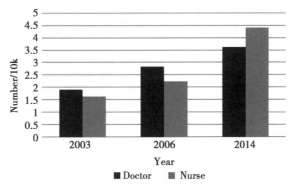

Fig.4-2   The number of ophthalmologists and
nurses in 2003,2006 and 2014

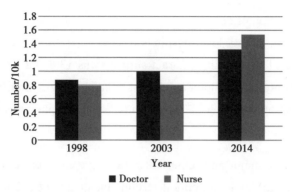

Fig.4-3   The number of ophthalmologists and nurses
in county-level hospitals in 1998,2003 and 2014

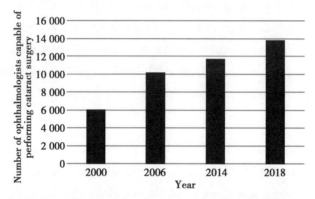

Fig.4-4   The number of ophthalmologists capable of
performing cataract surgery in 2000,2006,2014,and 2018

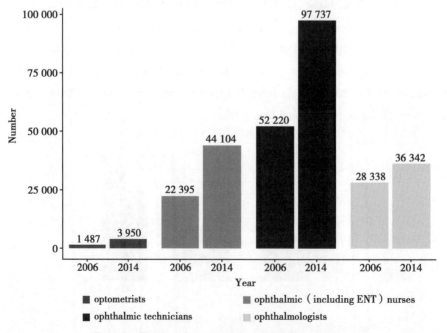

Fig.4-5   The number of ophthalmologists,nurses,
and optometrists in 2006 and 2014

III. Gradual improvement of equipping of ophthalmic equipment

In 2016, Chinese government launched the *Basic Standard for Medical Service Capacity of County-Level Hospitals* and *Recommended Standard for Medical Service Capacity of County-Level Hospitals* (GWBYF [2016] No. 12), which clearly stated the medical techniques and devices and equipment that clinical departments of county-level hospitals, including the ophthalmology department, should possess. Ophthalmic equipment, as an important part of ophthalmic resources, plays a key role in the improvement of primary eye care services. With the number of ophthalmic institutions and professionals in county-level hospitals increased, the equipping rate of ophthalmic equipment has also been improved. The equipping rates of non-contact tonometers, ophthalmic A/B ultrasound scanners, phaco emulsifiers and surgical microscopes have increased significantly. In 2015, more than 80% of county-level hospitals were equipped with non-contact tonometers, surgical microscopes, direct ophthalmoscopes and indirect ophthalmoscopes. Nearly half of the county-level hospitals were equipped with phaco emulsifiers and perimeters [1, 11] (Table 4-1, Fig.4-6).

Table 4-1.   Comparison of equipping rates of ophthalmic equipments in 2003 and 2015

Year	Ophthalmoto-nometer/%	Indirect ophthal-moscope/%	Direct ophthal-moscope/%	Ophthalmic A/B ultrasound/%	Phacoe-mulsifier/%	Surgical micro-scope/%	Perimeter/%
2003	80.9	39.8	63.5	25.7	12.1	61.0	33.1
2015	89.6	42.9	84.2	76.0	44.4	83.4	40.7

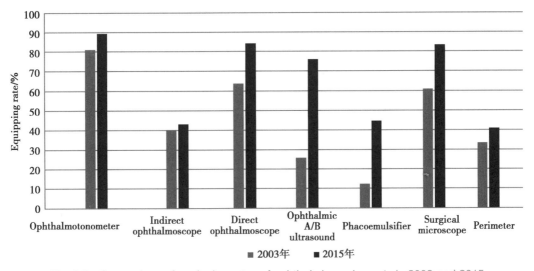

Fig.4-6   Comparison of equipping rates of ophthalmic equipments in 2003 and 2015

Chapter IV   Ophthalmic Resources

References

1. WANG Y. Statistical Analysis Report on the Status of Ophthalmology in China (2003)[Z]. 2004.

2. FENG JJ, AN LEI, WANG ZHIFENG, et al. Analysis on ophthalmic human resource allocation and service delivery at county level in Mainland China in 2014 [J]. Chinese journal of ophthalmology, 2018, 054 (012): 929-934.

3. ZHAN L, SAFAYA N, ERKOU H, et al. A comparative analysis on human resources among the specialized ophthalmic institutions in China [J]. Human resources for health, 2020, 18 (1).

4. ZHANG WB, LIU JJ. Evaluation of ophthalmological hygienic resonrces and utilized efficancy of healthy service in the county-ievel hospitals of China [J]. Medicine and society, 2001, 014 (006): 57-59.

5. XU HF, ZHANG WB. Present condition of ophthalmology resource in China in 2000%[J]. Medicine and society, 2005, 018 (005): 7-9.

6. National Bureau of Statistics. Statistical communique of the People's Republic of China on the 2017 national economic and social development.[ED/OL].(2018-02-28)[2020-04-15]. http://www. stats. gov. cn/tjsj/zxfb/201802/t20180228_1585631. html.

7. THYLEFORS B. A global initiative for the elimination of avoidable blindness [J]. Community eye health, 1998, 11 (25): 1-3.

8. JING ZW, REN H, WANG HY, et al. Analysis of human resources allocation of ophthalmic nurses in China [J]. Modern nursing, 2019, 25 (6): 703-707.

9. World Health Organization. Universal eye health: a global action plan 2014-2019.(2013-05-24)[2020-04-19]. https://apps. who. int/iris/bitstream/handle/10665/105937/9789245506560_chi. pdf; jsessionid=938CF4336F6ED37306821D82CE8076BB? sequence=9.

10. Publicity Department of National Health Commission of the People's Republic of China.[People's Daily] The overall myopia rate in children and adolescents reaches 53.6%, China will hold more targeted interventions.[EB/OL].(2019-05-08)[2020-04-15]. http://www. nhc. gov. cn/xcs/s7847/201905/11c679a40eb3494cade977f65f1c3740. shtml.

11. LIAO P, XU X, JING ZW, et al. Analysis of county hospitals'ophthalmic equipment configuration in China [J]. Chinese hospital management, 2019 39 (04): 62-65.

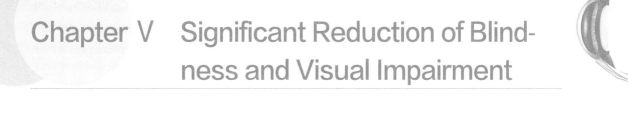

Chapter V Significant Reduction of Blindness and Visual Impairment

At the 2016 National Health Conference, Xi Jinping, general secretary of the Communist Party of China Central Committee, emphasized that strategic priority should be given to the people's health. Eye health is an important part of physical and mental health, but currently, blindness and visual impairment are still seriously affecting people's eye health. The Second China National Sample Survey on Disability in 2006 showed that the number of visually impaired people was 12.33 million[1], accounting for 14.86% of the total number of the disabled in China.

Over the years, under the leadership of the National Health Commission, and by virtue of the technical support of the National Committee for the Prevention of Blindness, and continuous efforts of blindness prevention personnel at all levels, China has been persistently engaging in the prevention and treatment of blindness by the following measures:(1) Hold various publicity activities based on dissemination activities on National Eye Care Day, World Sight Day and World Glaucoma Week, etc. to improve the public awareness of self-care; organize the compilation and publication of books for blindness prevention at primary level facilities and publicity materials for blindness prevention education; conduct diversified publicity and education activities on the prevention and treatment of blindness via newspapers, radio, television, and the Internet, to raise awareness among the public. (2) Vigorously promote the tradition of "Virtual of Great Physicians, Heal the Wounded and Rescue the Dying", report the vivid stories of ophthalmologists and primary medical staff treating eye diseases for the poor, and create a good public atmosphere of actively participating in the work of prevention and treatment of blindness. (3) Attach importance to the sight restoration for cataract patients, especially the poor, and treat millions of patients in remote areas through various blindness prevention and treatment projects. (4) Construct a relatively comprehensive ophthalmic medical service network suited to the reality in China depending on the projects, such as "Standardized Training to Elevate Eyecare in Rural China", so as to improve the blindness prevention and treatment system and provide overall, equal, and accessible ophthalmic medical services for Chinese people. (5) Persistently strengthen and promote the cooperation and exchanges between various areas by virtue of the network of the committees of the prevention of blindness at the national, provincial (autonomous regions and municipalities directly under the central government) and municipal level, to persistently summarize the experience in blindness prevention and treatment, such as the exchange of experience in blindness prevention through eye health newsletters, publications and regular regional or national conferences. (6) Train backbone staff in various provinces (autonomous regions and municipalities directly under the central government), cities, and regions through regularly organizing national workshops or training courses.

Based on all these efforts, the prevention and control of blindness and visual impairment in China have made great progress. The health authorities led two epidemiological surveys on blindness and visual impairment in nine provinces (autonomous regions and municipalities directly under the central government) in 2006 and 2014 respectively, and the assessment based on the best corrected visual acuity showed that the prevalence of moderate to severe visual impairment in people over 50 decreased from 10.8% in 2006 to 10.3% in 2014, decreasing by 4.6%; in addition, the blindness rate decreased from 2.29% in 2006 to 1.66% in 2014, decreasing by 27.5% [2]. Based on the census data in 2010, it could be estimated that blindness was prevented in a million people over 50. The surveys indicated that the prevalence of blindness and visual impairment has significantly decreased, and great progress has been made in the work of prevention and treatment of blindness in China.

References

1. National Bureau of Statistics of People's Republic of China. Data bulletin of the second China national sample survey on disability in 2006 [EB/OL].(2006-12-01)[2020-06-17]. http://www. gov. cn/ztzl/gacjr/content_459223. htm.
2. ZHAO J, XU X, ELLWEIN LB, et al. Causes of visual impairment and blindness in the 2006 and 2014 nine-province surveys in rural China [J]. Am J Ophthalmol, 2019, 197: 80-87.

Chapter VI Changes in Spectrum of Major Blinding Eye Diseases

With the advancement of blindness prevention work, the improvement of the economic level, and the change in people's lifestyle and demographic structure, significant changes have taken place in the spectrum of leading blinding eye diseases. The leading blinding eye diseases have changed from infectious eye diseases, such as trachoma, to metabolic and age-related non-infectious eye diseases, such as cataract, keratopathy, retinal diseases, refractive error, glaucoma, and amblyopia.

I. Cataract

During the "13th 5-Year Plan " period, the cataract surgical rate (CSR) and percentage of patients with postoperative vision >0.3 were significantly improved, but with China entering an aging society, the demand of the elderly for eye care would increase significantly. People over 40 are at high risk for age-related eye diseases, including cataract, with a prevalence of 50% in people aged 60~69, which further increases to 79.2% in people over 70[1]. In 2017, the population over 60 (including) reached 241 million in China, accounting for 17.3% of the total population[2], which, as estimated, will reach 480 million by 2050. In the elderly population with high disease prevalence, high disability rate and high medical service utilization rate, eye health problems will become prominent. At present, cataract is still the leading blinding eye disease in China, therefore, the main task of prevention and treatment of blindness is to improve CSR, increase surgical coverage, and ensure better surgical quality.

II. Keratopathy

In China, keratopathy is the second most common blinding eye disease, following cataract. In addition, the blinding risk of keratopathy is higher than that of other eye diseases, reaching over 70% [3]. The work of eye health in China, especially when infectious keratopathy is involved, should focus on the diagnosis and treatment of keratopathy and the prevention of corneal blindness.

In recent years, the source of cornea donation has been broadened in China. In addition to the traditional donation source, the corneal lamellar materials left from laser myopia surgery and artificial corneal materials were also used. At present, there may be nearly 10,000 patients recovering sight through corneal transplantation every year [4], and the figure was only 1,000 in the 1990s. However, considering the number of patients, the demand has not been fully met. In the future, the prevention and treatment of corneal blindness will still focus on expanding the sources of cornea donation and training specialists for treating keratopathy.

III. Retinal diseases such as maculopathy and diabetic retinopathy

With the continuous improvement of people's living standard and the changes in lifestyles, the incidence of chronic diseases is increasing year by year; therefore, the number of patients suffering from the related fundus diseases, such as hypertensive fundus disease, diabetic retinopathy, and age-related macular degeneration, is also increasing greatly. Due to the complicated etiology and long duration, fundus diseases have gradually become a major cause of irreversible blindness.

Early screening and interventions are effective for fundus diseases. Diabetic retinopathy is known as the leading preventable blinding fundus disease, and blindness and visual impairment caused by diabetic retinopathy can be effectively avoided through early screening, regular follow-up, and timely laser treatment. The wide application of anti-vascular endothelial growth factor (anti-VEGF) can delay the progression of the disease and the visual function could be partly restored. At present, Ranibizumab, Aflibercept, Conbercept and other anti-VEGF drugs have been included in the basic medical insurance directory. The collected data showed that there is one diabetic patient in every ten adults over 20 [5]. The high prevalence of diabetes indicates a high prevalence of diabetic retinopathy and the large number of patients with blindness caused by diabetic retinopathy. The statistics showed that the prevalence of diabetic retinopathy was 1.3% in the general population in China [6]. In the future, the screening of fundus diseases will be the focus of eye health work. At present, many institutions have carried out screening, for example, the National Committee for the Prevention of Blindness and the Chinese Society of Microcirculation have organized " China Diabetic Retinopathy Screening and Prevention Project " for "improving the screening rate of diabetic retinopathy and avoiding blindness in diabetic patients". As of November 2019, the China Diabetic Retinopathy Screening and Prevention Project has covered 577 hospitals (including more than 200 tertiary hospitals) in 29 provinces (autonomous regions and municipalities directly under the central government), and more than 800,000 diabetic patients have been screened.

IV. Refractive error

Myopia is one of the most common types of refractive error. The high myopia-induced complications can result in low vision and even blindness. In some regions in China, retinopathy related to high myopia has become the primary cause of irreversible blinding eye diseases in adults. Therefore, the prevention and treatment of myopia have been highlighted in eye health work in China. The survey showed that the overall rate of myopia has reached 53.6% in children and adolescents [7] and over 90% in college students in certain areas [8], and the prevalence of high myopia has reached over 10% [8,9]. In addition, uncorrected moderate to high hyperopia and astigmatism can also affect the normal visual development of children, and thus resulting in strabismus and amblyopia, and affecting the development of the normal visual function.

The easiest way to resolve the issue caused by refractive error is to wear properly fitted glasses. In China, great efforts have been made to tackle blindness and visual impairment caused by refractive error through cultivating human resources for optometry services and providing high-quality and inexpensive glasses, as well as convenient and accessible optometry services.

V. Glaucoma

In China, the prevalence of glaucoma reaches up to 2.58%, and the number of glaucoma patients, as estimated, will reach 25.16 million by 2020 [10]. The onset of glaucoma is acute and its pathogenesis remains unclear, thus there is no etiological treatment. Clinically, the cause of glaucoma is latent and complicated in most patients, therefore, the treatment is often delayed. Especially for the primary open-angle glaucoma, it is hard to diagnose and detect at an early stage. Most patients may have already had obvious optic nerve damage upon initial diagnosis. Hence, there is a high blinding rate. In recent years, with the continuous promotion of appropriate techniques in China, the blinding rate of glaucoma has significantly decreased compared with that in the 1990s, and the blinding rate of acute angle-closure glaucoma has decreased from 50% [11] in the 1990s to 14.5% in recent years. The detection rate of open-angle glaucoma has increased from 10% to 40%.

Considering that the blindness caused by glaucoma is irreversible and due to the lack of awareness among the public, the publicity and education activities should be strengthened, so as to achieve early detection and early treatment. In addition, glaucoma should be considered as one of the key contents for the training of physicians in primary hospitals. Most primary hospitals lack glaucoma specialists, and glaucoma is mainly treated with trabeculectomy, which has a relatively poor long-term effect. In addition, some patients are not followed up in a standardized way, thereby failing to avoid blindness. Therefore, while emphasizing early detection and strengthening screening, all hospitals should also focus on the standardized follow-up, especially for primary open-angle glaucoma and chronic angle-closure glaucoma. In the future, the training of glaucoma should be organized for primary ophthalmologists, which should focus on the use of fundus photography, perimetry and optical coherence tomography in the standardized follow-up of glaucoma patients in addition to measurement of intraocular pressure. Since 2017, for three consecutive years, the theme of "World Glaucoma Week" stressed the importance of fundus examination. In the future, the prevention and treatment of glaucoma focusing on community-based screening for high-risk population of glaucoma by means of artificial intelligence will become the priority.

VI. Amblyopia

In China, the prevalence of amblyopia is about 2.8% in children aged 3 to 6 and about 3.5% in those aged 6 to 14. Childhodd is a critical and sensitive period for visual development, and the screening of amblyopia-related risk factors, such as strabismus, refractive error, and anisometropia, is the key to early detection and treatment of amblyopia. In 2013, for detecting the eye diseases that may affect the visual development of children, realizing early correction and timely referral, preventing the occurrence and development of controllable eye diseases, and protecting and promoting normal development of visual function in children, the national health administrations issued the *Technical Specifications for Eye and Vision Care for Children*, which clearly stipulated that children should regularly receive the screening of eye diseases and vision assessment and pay attention to eye health habits, so as to prevent eye traumas and infectious eye diseases [12-14].

Several projects have been organized in China, including the national health industry special project "Study on Standardization and Application of Screening, Diagnosis and Intervention Techniques for Common Blinding Eye Diseases", Orbis International's major cooperation project "Epidemiological Study on Children Strabismus, Amblyopia and Refractive Error in Tianjin and Yunnan", and other population-based large-sample epidemiological surveys on strabismus, amblyopia, and vision development in children. In addition, after discussion by experts on strabismus and pediatric ophthalmology at several conferences, the *Expert Consensus on Diagnosis of Amblyopia* was launched, with which, the unnecessary waste of medical resources due to expanded diagnosis of amblyopia in preschool children and excessive diagnosis and treatment has gradually decreased. Nevertheless, due to the high prevalence of amblyopia up to 3% [15], early detection and intervention of amblyopia will still be the key to the prevention and treatment of blindness and low vision in children.

References

1. YUAN X B, ZHANG D Y, CHEN S J, et al. Prevalence of cataract among the population aged 50 years and over at different altitudes in Gansu Province [J]. Zhonghua yan ke za zhi, 2019, 55 (8): 589-594.

2. China National Blindness Prevention and Treatment. Ranking of cataract surgery reports in China in 2017. [EB/OL].(2018-03-28)[2020-05-13]. http://www. moheyes. com/News/Details/3bed4465-7e8c-40e3-8532-25eeb128565b.

3. GAO H, CHEN X N, SHI W Y. Analysis of the prevalence of blindness and major blinding diseases in China [J]. Chinese journal of ophthalmology, 2019, 55 (8): 625-628.

4. SHI W Y, XIE L X. The status quo and expectation of corneal research in China [J]. Chinese journal of ophthalmology, 2014, 50 (9): 641-645.

5. YANG W, LU J, WENG J, et al. Prevalence of diabetes among men and women in China [J]. N Engl j med, 2010, 362 (12): 1090-1101.

6. Fundus Ophthalmology Group of Ophthalmology Branch, Chinese Medical Association. Guidelines for clinical diagnosis and treatment of diabetic retinopathy in China (2014)[J]. Chinese journal of ophthal-mology, 2014, 50 (11): 851-865.

7. Department of Publicity of National Health Commission of People's Republic of China.[EB/OL].(2019-05-08) [2020-04-15]. http://www. nhc. gov. cn/xcs/s7847/201905/11c679a40eb3494cade977f65f1c3740. shtml.

8. DONG L, KANG Y K, LI Y, et al. Prevalence and time trends of myopia in children and adolescents in China: a systemic review and meta-analysis [J]. Retina. 2020, 40 (3): 399-411.

9. SUN J, ZHOU J, ZHAO P, et al. High prevalence of myopia and high myopia in 5060 Chinese university students in Shanghai [J]. Invest ophthalmol vis sci, 2012, 53: 7504-7509.

10. SONG P, WANG J, BUCAN K, et al. National and subnational prevalence and burden of glaucoma in China: a systematic analysis [J]. J glob health, 2017, 7 (2): 20705.

11. LI H M. Investigation on blindness rate of primary glaucoma in rural areas in Xiangtan [J]. Hunan medical journal, 1986, 03: 158.

12. ZHAO K X. Early diagnosis and prompt intervention for launching a fruitful campaign against ambly-opia [J]. Chinese journal of ophthalmology, 2002, 38 (8): 449-451.

13. ZHAO K X, ZHENG Y Z. Problems to be resolved urgently on amblyopia diagnosis and prevention in China [J]. Chinese journal of ophthalmology, 2009, 45 (11): 961-962.

14. ZHAO K X, SHI X F. Pay attention to abnormal vision screening for infants and young children [J]. Chinese journal of ophthalmology, 2013, 49 (7): 577-579.

15. Bureau of Medical Administration of National Health Commission of People's Republic of China. Ambly-opia is a serious and avoidable visual impairment disease, and there are about 40 million amblyopia patients in China.[EB/OL].(2018-06-05)[2020-05-19]. http://www. nhc. gov. cn/yzygj/s7652/201806/f8477829bfe 149aebe4d75ddce0a663e. shtml.

Chapter VII   Prevention and Control of Myopia

I. Current situation of myopia in children and adolescents

Refractive error, one of the major causes of visual impairment around the world, was listed as one of the five major eye diseases that lead to avoidable blindness and visual impairment and to be eliminated [1,2], while myopic refractive error is the primary cause of uncorrected visual impairment [3]. According to statistics, the number of myopic patients will reach 4.758 billion by 2050, accounting for 49.8% of the world's population [4]. In recent years, with the economic and social development and aggravation of intellectual competition, the prevalence of myopia in children and adolescents has maintained high in China, indicating the characteristics of "Early onset age, rapid increase of prevalence, rapid progression and high degree of myopia", therefore, it has become an important public health issue affecting eye health of Chinese children and adolescents.

As surveyed in different regions across China, the prevalence of myopia varies across ages and regions. The survey on preschool children in Shanghai showed that the prevalence of myopia in children aged 4, 5 and 6 reached 2.3%, 3.5% and 5.2%, respectively [5]. In elementary and middle school students, the prevalence increased significantly. The survey in Guangzhou showed that the average prevalence of myopia in students of Grade 1-9 reached 47.4%, and the prevalence of myopia increased from 0.2% in Grade 1 to 68.4% in Grade 9,(48.9% in Han students and 35.6% in students of other ethnic groups) [6]. The survey in Anyang, Henan Province, showed that the prevalence of myopia in students of Grade 1 and Grade 7 reached 3.9% and 67.3%, respectively [7], while that in college students reached 83.2%, of which, the prevalence of high myopia has reached 11.1% [8].

In addition, the Handan Eye Study showed that the prevalence of myopia in people over 30 was 26.7% and the prevalence of high myopia was only 1.8% [9]. Compared with the prevalence of myopia among adults, the prevalence of myopia among children and adolescents is much higher, indicating markedly increased myopia prevalence in this generation.

In the second half of 2018, the National Health Commission, together with Ministry of Education and Ministry of Civil Affairs, organized a national survey on myopia in children and adolescents, which involved 1,117,400 students in 1,033 kindergartens and 3,810 elementary and secondary schools. On April 29, 2019, the National Health Commission held a press conference and released the results of the survey on myopia in children and adolescents in 2018, indicating that the overall myopia rate in children and adolescents was 53.6% in 2018 [10], of which 14.5% in children aged 6, 36.0% in elementary school students, 71.6% in junior high school students, and 81.0% in senior high school students. In addition, the problem of myopia was more prominent in younger children, as in the elementary and junior high school period, the myopia rate would increase rapidly with the increase of grade, increasing from 15.7% in Grade 1 to 59.0% in Grade 6 in elementary school period, and from 64.9% in Grade 1 to 77.0% in Grade 3 in junior high school period. In Grade 3 in senior high school period, the proportion of students suffering from high myopia (more than 6 diopters) reached 21.9% of total myopic students.

II. National strategy for prevention and control of myopia

In addition to inconveniences in daily life and study, myopia, especially high myopia, may also lead to several serious complications, such as glaucoma, cataract, retinal detachment, and macular degeneration [11]. Therefore, the prevention and treatment of myopia are taken as an important issue concerned by the Chinese government.

In recent years, the Central Committee of the Communist Party of China and State Council have attached great importance to the prevention and control of myopia in children and adolescents, which has been considered as a national strategy. From 2016 to 2019, the themes of National Eye Care Day focused on the prevention and control of myopia in children and adolescents for four consecutive years:"Take care of eyes since childhood", " Prevent myopia, and enjoy the sunshine " , " Scientifically prevent and control myopia, and take care of eye health of the children", and " Take good care of the children's eyes jointly, and ensure them a bright future " . On June 5, 2018, the National Health Commission held a press conference, which introduced the scientific prevention and control of myopia in children and adolescents. At the same time, it also launched the *Guidelines for Myopia Prevention*, *Guidelines for Amblyopia Prevention* and *Guidelines for Strabismus Prevention*, which aimed to guide medical institutions and eye care personnel to improve their ability to provide services and to guide the students and parents to establish correct awareness of eye care habits. In order to clarify the baseline prevalence of myopia in children and adolescents in various regions, the General Office of the National Health Commission, General Office of the Ministry of Education, and General Office of the Ministry of Finance jointly launched the *Notice on Carrying Out the Survey on Myopia in Children and Adolescents in 2018* (GWBJKH [2018] No. 932).

On August 28, 2018, Xi Jinping, general secretary of the Communist Party of China Central Committee, presented another important instruction and emphasized that the whole society should take good care of children's eyes, and provide them with a bright future. In order to implement General Secretary Xi's instruction and effectively strengthen the prevention and control of myopia in children and adolescents in the new era, the Ministry of Education, together with the National Health Commission, the General Administration of Sport of China, the Ministry of Finance, the Ministry of Human Resources and Social Security, the State Administration for Market Regulation, National Press and Publication Administration, and National Radio and Television Administration, launched the *Implementation Plan for Comprehensive Prevention and Control of Myopia in Children and Adolescents* [12] (JTY [2018] No. 3)(hereinafter referred to as the *Implementation Plan*) on August 30, 2018. The *Implementation Plan* clarified the prevention and control measures that should be taken by the families, schools, medical and health institutions, students, and the related government departments, as well as responsibilities and tasks of the eight ministries and commissions for the prevention and control of myopia. In addition, it also emphasized that the directors of the people's governments at the provincial level should personally engage in the prevention and control of myopia. The national evaluation and assessment system for the prevention and control of myopia in children and adolescents should be established, to clarify the prevalence of myopia in children and adolescents in various regions in 2018, and in 2019, all provincial governments should be evaluated, and the results should be publicized.

In 2019, the National Health Commission, together with the Ministry of Education, organized a series of publicity activities on the theme of "prevention of myopia in children and adolescents" , which improved the health literacy of children and adolescents. The Bureau of Disease Prevention and Control of National Health Commission prepared and issued the *Guidelines for Suitable Techniques for Prevention and Treatment of Myopia in Children and Adolescents*, so as to guide the scientific and standardized prevention and control of myopia and improve the technical capabilities for prevention and control. The General Office of the Ministry of Education issued the *Notice on Publishing the Selection Results of Pilot Counties* (*Cities, Districts*) *and Reform Pilot Areas for Prevention and Treatment of Myopia in Children and Adolescents* (JTYTH [2018] No. 77), which named 84 regions, such as Dongcheng District of Beijing, as the pilot counties (cities, districts), and 29 pilot reform areas for the prevention and control of myopia in children and adolescents, such as Beichen District of Tianjin. The National Committee for the Prevention of Blindness compiled the *100 Questions on Popularization of Prevention and*

Treatment of Myopia in Children and Adolescents, which scientifically explained the questions and misunderstandings in the prevention and treatment of myopia. In addition, for realizing scientific prevention and control and precise implementation of policies, the Bureau of Disease Prevention and Control of National Health Commission and Beijing Tongren Hospital, Capital Medical University (hereinafter referred to as Beijing Tongren Hospital) jointly prepared the *Manual of Myopia Prevention and Control in Kindergartens*, *Manual of Myopia Prevention and Control in Primary School Students*, *Manual of Myopia Prevention and Control in Junior Middle School Students*, and *Manual of Myopia Prevention and Control in Senior Middle School Students* for children and adolescents in different age groups. At present, a good atmosphere of " leadership by government, cooperation among sectors, guidance by experts, education in school, commitment in family " for the prevention and control of myopia in children and adolescents has been formed in the society.

III. Comprehensive prevention and control measures

In view of the characteristics of myopia in children and adolescents, various measures have been taken to realize comprehensive prevention and control of myopia in China, such as the strict implementation of the requirements for eye health and vision examination in children aged 0 to 6 in basic public health services, and the establishment of refractive development files, so as to realize early monitoring, early detection, early warning, and early intervention. The diagnosis and treatment should be standardized, and general hospitals at county level and above should provide ophthalmic medical services, and earnestly implement the *Guidelines for Myopia Prevention* and other diagnosis and treatment specifications, so as to persistently improve the capabilities of providing eye care services. They should strengthen health education, myopia screening and census of myopia in elementary and secondary school students, and initiate the children and adolescents, as well as their parents, to autonomously engage in health actions. Moreover, they should actively engage in the research related to prevention and treatment of myopia, strengthen the application and comprehensive promotion of the achievements and techniques for prevention and treatment of myopia.

Considering the impact of multiple environmental factors on the development and progression of myopia, such as the lack of outdoor activities, excessive use of electronic products, and unhealthy eye habits, the schools and parents should add outdoor activities and exercises, guide children and adolescents to engage in outdoor activities or physical exercises, and control the use of electronic products, avoid unhealthy eye habits, and guide children and adolescents to maintain the distance of " one chi (=1/3 metre), one fist, and one cun (=1/3 decimetre)" during reading [13]. Teaching activities should be arranged in strict accordance with the national curriculum plan and standards, and the parents should reasonably select extracurricular trainings for their children based on hobbies rather than blindly ask them to participate in such trainings. All children should keep doing eye exercises

Chapter Ⅶ Prevention and Control of Myopia

and ensure sufficient sleep and nutrition. As for the children with myopia, scientific diagnosis and treatment, as well as correction, should be adopted, such as the wearing of glasses or orthokeratology lenses, the use of low-concentration atropine, etc [14].

References

1. PASCOLINI D, MARIOTTI S. Global estimates of visual impairment: 2010 [J]. Br j ophthalmol, 2012, 96 (5): 614-618.
2. ZHAO J, XU X, ELLWEIN L, et al. Prevalence of vision impairment in older adults in rural China in 2014 and comparisons with the 2006 China nine-province survey [J]. am j ophthalmol, 2018, 185 (1): 81-93.
3. XU L, WANG Y, LI Y, et al. Causes of blindness and visual impairment in urban and rural areas in Beijing: the Beijing eye study [J]. Ophthalmology, 2006, 113 (7): 1134-1137.
4. HOLDEN B, FRICKE T, WILSON D, et al. Global prevalence of myopia and high myopia and temporal trends from 2000 through 2050 [J]. Ophthalmology, 2016, 123 (5): 1036-1042.
5. MA Y, QU X, ZHU X, et al. Age-specific prevalence of visual impairment and refractive error in children aged 3-10 years in Shanghai, China [J]. Invest ophthalmol vis sci, 2016, 57 (14): 6188-6196.
6. GUO L, YANG J, MAI J, et al. Prevalence and associated factors of myopia among primary and middle school-aged students: a school-based study in Guangzhou [J]. Eye, 2016, 30 (6): 796-804.
7. LI S, LIU L, LI S, et al. Design, methodology and baseline data of a school-based cohort study in central China: the Anyang Childhood Eye Study [J]. Ophthalmic epidemiol, 2013, 20 (6): 348-359.
8. WEI S, SUN Y, LI S, et al. Refractive errors in university students in central China: the Anyang university students eye study [J]. Invest ophthalmol vis sci, 2018, 59 (11): 4691-4700.
9. LIANG Y, WONG T, SUN L, et al. Refractive errors in a rural Chinese adult population the Handan eye study [J]. Ophthalmology, 2009, 116 (11): 2119-2127.
10. Department of Publicity of National Health Commission of People's Republic of China. The overall myopia rate of children and adolescents is 53.6%, China will carry out more targeted myopia intervention.(2019-05-08)[2020-04-15]. http://www. nhc. gov. cn/xcs/s7847/201905/11c679a40eb3494cade977f65f1c3740. shtml.
11. SAW S, GAZZARD G, SHIH-YEN E, et al. Myopia and associated pathological complications [J]. Ophthalmic physiol opt, 2005, 25 (5): 381-391.
12. Ministry of Education of People's Republic of China, National Health Commission of People's Republic of China, General Administration of Sport of China, et al. Notice on Issuing the Implementation Plan for Comprehensive Prevention and Treatment of Myopia in Children and Adolescents by Eight Ministres/Commissions [EB/OL].(2018-08-30)[2020-04-05]. http://www. moe. gov. cn/srcsite/A17/moe_943/s3285/201808/t20180830_346672. html.
13. LI S, LI S, KANG M, et al. Near work related parameters and myopia in Chinese children: the Anyang childhood eye study [J]. Plos one, 2015, 10 (8): e0134514.
14. WALLINE J, LINDSLEY K, VEDULA S, et al. Interventions to slow progression of myopia in children [J]. Cochrane database syst rev, 2020, 1: CD004916.

Chapter VIII Elimination of Blinding Trachoma

I. High prevalence of trachoma in the 1950s

Around the founding of the People's Republic of China, trachoma was the leading cause of blindness, and almost "nine out of ten people had trachoma". The statistics by occupations indicated that the prevalence of trachoma was about 40%~70% in workers, 40%~80% in farmers, and 30%~70% in students; while the statistics by regions indicated that the prevalence of trachoma was about 30%~50% in the south of the Yangtze River and coastal areas, 40%~70% in the north of the Yangtze River and south of the Great Wall, 50%~80% in the northeastern area, and higher in Lanzhou and Xinjiang (60%~90%). The prevalence of vision impairment due to trachoma was about 55.8%, and the prevalence of blindness due to trachoma was about 7%, summing to 62.8%. [1]

II. Comprehensive prevention and treatment, scientific research, and remarkable progress

In the 1950s, the control of trachoma, the leading blinding eye disease, was incorporated in the national public health plan. In 1956, the prevention and treatment of trachoma was classified as one of the 60 tasks in the National Development Program which was released on October 1957. From 1957 to 1959, China made further efforts to prevent and treat trachoma and transform toilets, aiming to cut off the route of transmission of trachoma [1]. In 1958, the *National Trachoma Prevention and Treatment Plan* [2] was launched, which required promoting the hygiene-centered comprehensive prevention and treatment measures in combination with the "Patriotic Health Campaign". Specific measures were defined, such as the advocating "one towel for one person, and keep the towel clean", promoting face washing with running water, and changing the habit of washing face with the same basin or even the same basin of water in a family, paying attention to the protection of eyes, avoiding rubbing eyes with hands, and frequently washing hands and face, as well as the improvement of water quality, and maintaining the water clean. In addition, the sanitation of service industries was asked to be strictly supervised and the management strengthened. The awareness of collective prevention was asked to be improved in collective living units such as factories, schools and nurseries, to prevent and control the transmission of trachoma. At the same time, the government also proposed that trachoma must be controlled based on integration of prevention and treatment, which was a comprehensive measure to deal with trachoma. All institutions should strengthen the publicity and education on trachoma prevention and health education, and conduct regular publicity and education, so as to teach the public the measures for prevention and treatment of trachoma.

In view of the unknown pathogen, trachoma was once called the "dark region in ophthalmology"[3] In order to effectively prevent and treat trachoma, all ophthalmology staff actively responded to the call of the government and engaged in the prevention and treatment of trachoma. In August 1955, Professor Feifan Tang and Professor Xiaolou Zhang successfully isolated "Chlamydia trachomatis", the pathogen of trachoma for the first time in the world, greatly promoting the research and prevention of trachoma and being awarded the gold medal by the International Organization against Trachoma. Later, domestic scholars continued the etiological research on Chlamydia trachomatis, as well as pathogenic mechanism, local immunity, transmission route, therapeutic drugs and preventive measures from the perspective of clinical treatment and prevention. In addition, they also initiated the development of vaccines, and screened effective drugs, and thus made a major breakthrough in the prevention and treatment of trachoma[4].

The First China National Sample Survey on Disability in 1987 showed that the visual disability rate caused by trachoma was 102.01/100,000, accounting for 14.25% in visual disabilities (1,611/11,300); the blindness rate of trachoma was 46.98/100,000; and the low vision rate of trachoma was 55.02/100,000. The Survey indicated that the disability rate of trachoma accounted for 14.25% in visual disabilities, ranking the third[5].

Since the 1990s, National Committee for the Prevention of Blindness has been promoting the simplified grading standard and comprehensive trachoma prevention and treatment strategy of the WHO- "SAFE" Strategy: Surgery for Trichiasis (S), Antibiotic Treatment (A), Face Washing (F), Environmental Improvement (E). The Committee has also incorporated the education on trachoma prevention in textbooks for primary schools in combination with toilet transformation and "Patriotic Health Campaign", and created the SAFE model with Chinese characteristics, thus providing an effective and feasible method to eliminate blinding trachoma[6].

III. Achieving the goal of eliminating blinding trachoma in advance under the "VISION 2020" initiative

The elimination of blinding trachoma is one of the major goals of "VISION 2020: The Right to Sight "[7]. In 1999, the WHO estimated that China had the world's most trachoma patients due to the largest population, accounting for 1/4-1/3 of trachoma patients in the world, and about 6 million trichiasis patients needed to be treated by surgery. China's action is of great significance in eliminating blinding trachoma in the world. In 2003, Chinese representatives participated in the Meeting of the WHO Alliance for the Global Elimination of Blinding Trachoma in Geneva. The WHO estimated that there were 26 million patients with active trachoma (follicular trachoma and invasive trachoma), and 3 million with trachomatous trichiasis in China[8].

The Second China National Sample Survey on Disability in 2006 showed that the visual disability rate of trachoma was 17.62/100,000, accounting for 1.87% of visual disabilities. The blindness rate of trachoma was 7.84/100,000, and low vision rate of trachoma was 10.17/100,000 (fig. 8-1, fig. 8-2)[9]. Due to the lack of data, the evaluation on the elimination of blinding trachoma was conducted in 15 provinces (autonomous region and municipalities directly under the central government) in China from 2004 to 2007. Trachoma screening was provided for 59,630 children under 10, which found that the positive rate of follicular trachoma was 0.94%, and the screening for 82,434 adults over 50 showed that the positive rate of trachomatous trichiasis was 0.34%. These two surveys proved that, by virtue of continuous efforts of the Chinese government in improving public health environment and medical conditions, the prevalence of trachoma in China has significantly decreased from 30% in urban areas and 80% in rural areas in the 1950s, and the prevalence of trachoma in different regions has decreased to 2%-29%[10].

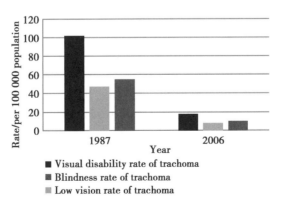

Fig.8-1   Comparison of visual disability caused by
trachoma in 1987 and 2006[11]

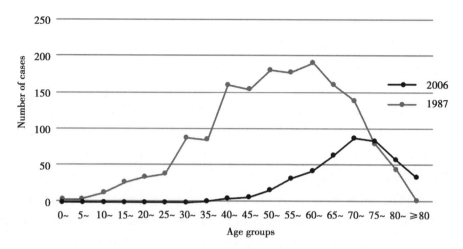

Fig.8-2 Distribution of visual disability cases caused by trachoma
by age groups in 1987 and 2006 [11]

For further confirming the progress in trachoma prevention and treatment, the National Committee for the Prevention of Blindness submitted an evaluation report on the elimination of blinding trachoma in China, and proposed to the national health administrations and Lions Clubs International to discuss the project plan. In September 2012, Phase III of " Sight First, China Action" - " Eliminate blinding trachoma in China by 2016 " was launched in Beijing, which was led by the Chinese government, funded by Lions Clubs International, participated by blindness prevention personnel of the WHO, and promoted by all governmental and medical administrations, management personnel, eye care personnel and disabled persons' federations in 31 provinces (autonomous regions and municipalities directly under the central government). The project " Eliminate blinding trachoma in China by 2016 " also focused on the screening, treatment and evaluation of trachoma. In areas suspected for high prevalence of trachoma, rapid assessment of trachoma was conducted. The project covered 31 provinces (autonomous regions and municipalitiesdirectly under the central government and autonomous regions) in China. Baseline assessment of trachoma and patient intervention were implemented in 16 provinces (autonomous regions and municipalitiesdirectly under the central government and autonomous regions), and the epidemiological survey in 130 primary schools and 55,679 villages in these 16 provinces (autonomous regions and municipalitiesdirectly under the central government and autonomous regions) showed that the prevalence of active trachoma and trachomatous trichiasis was 0.196% and 0.002%, respectively, indicating that there was no trachoma-endemic areas in China, and even in areas suffering from water shortage, the prevalence of active trachoma was lower than 5%, and that of trachomatous trichiasis was lower than 0.1%. In addition, 16 patients with active trachoma and 1,334 with trachomatous trichiasis were treated in the project [12-13].

Ⅳ. Summary

Public health and medical conditions in China have been greatly improved by virtue of the long-term investment and efforts of the Chinese government, as well as the measures of providing education on trachoma prevention among the young, incorporating "frequent washing of hands and face" and "one towel for one person" in textbooks for elementary schools, promoting toilet transformation, Patriotic Health Campaign and environmental improvement, economic and medical development, and investment in rural medical construction and medical insurance. The availability of antibiotics for trachoma patients was greatly improved, and the implementation of SAFE strategy was vigorously promoted. Therefore, the work of trachoma prevention and treatment in China was affirmed and praised at the ninth meeting of the WHO Alliance for the Global Elimination of Blinding Trachoma [14]. On May 18, 2015, the National Health and Family Planning Commission officially announced at the 68th World Health Assembly that China met the WHO's requirement for controlling blinding trachoma and eliminating blinding trachoma in advance [13], and thus trachoma was no longer a public health issue endangering vision health in China. On February 12, 2020, China received a letter from the WHO, which reviewed the documents provided by China in December 2019 and determined that trachoma was eliminated and removed from the list of public health issues in China. Later, the trachoma pandemic status on the page of Global Health Observatory was changed to the public health issue has been eliminated. The early elimination of blinding trachoma in China, with 1/5 of the world's population, will promote the development of hygiene and eye health in China, and will also be of great significance to the prevention and treatment of trachoma in the world. It has played a great promoting role in and made great contributions to the elimination of avoidable blindness worldwide.

───────── References ─────────

1. WANG N, HU A, TAYLOR H. Trachoma [M]. Beijng: People's Medical Publishing House, 2015: 24-25.
2. Abstract of national trachoma prevention and treatment plan (Amended Draft)[J]. Chinese journal of medicine, 1959.
3. JIN X. History and progress of study on chlamydia trachomatis [J]. Ophthalmology in China, 2006 (3).
4. WANG N, DENG S, TIAN L. A review of trachoma history in China: research, prevention, and control [J]. Science China life sciences, 2016, 59 (6): 541-547.
5. Office of China National Sample Survey on Disability. Data of China national sample survey on disability in 1987 [Z].

6. WANG N, HU A. Enlightenment and thinking of trachoma prevention and treatment in China [J]. Chinese journal of ophthalmology, 2015 (7): 484-486.

7. ZHAO J. "Vision 2020" and prevention of blindness in China [J]. Chinese journal of ophthalmology, 2002 (10): 4-6.

8. WANG N, HU A, HUGH R TAYLOR. Trachoma [M]. Beijng: People's Medical Publishing House, 2015: 37.

9. Office of the Second China National Sample Survey on Disability. Data of the second china national sample survey on disability [Z]. China statistics press. 2006.

10. WANG N, HU A, HUGH R TAYLOR. Trachoma [M]. Beijng: People's Medical Publishing House, 2015: 39.

11. HU A, CAI X, QIAO L, et al. Comparison of visual impairment caused by trachoma in China between 1978 and 2006 [J]. Chinese journal of ophthalmology, 2015, 51 (10): 768-772.

12. ZHAO J, MARIOTTI S, RESNIKOFF S, et al. Assessment of trachoma in suspected endemic areas within 16 provinces in mainland China [J]. Plos negl trop dis, 2019; 13 (1): e0007130.

13. WANG N, HU A, TAYLOR H. Trachoma [M]. Beijing: People's Medical Publishing House, 2015: 49-50.

14. World Health Organization, Report of the ninth meeting of the WHO alliance for the global elimination of blinding trachoma [C], 2005, 21.

Chapter IX   Low Vision Rehabilitation

Low vision is one of the major causes of avoidable blindness to be addressed under the VISION 2020 initiative. Chinese government made a commitment to eliminate avoidable blindness (including low vision) by 2020. In 2013, WHA passed a resolution, which adjusted the objective of "VISION 2020". It proposed the "Universal Eye Health: A Global Action Plan 2014-2019", aiming to reduce the avoidable visual impairment (a global public health issue) and enable the patients with visual impairment to enjoy various rehabilitation services. As a member state of "VISION 2020" declaration, China has been actively promoting the related work, and preparing and implementing the policies, plans and programs for visual impairment rehabilitation.

I. Initiation of low vision rehabilitation work in China

The low vision rehabilitation was not started until the early 1980s in China. In 1983, Beijing Tongren Hospital established the first outpatient department for low vision, which filled the gap of low vision rehabilitation service in China. The first training class of low vision was held in 1986, the first domestic typoscope was developed in 1986, the first monograph on low vision-*Clinical Low Vision*-was published in 1988, and the first textbook for higher education-*Low Vision*-was compiled in 2004. In addition, numerous low vision clinics were set nationwide, indicating the launch of low vision rehabilitation work throughout China.

II. Academic exchange in low vision rehabilitation

In order to stay updated on the major events of low vision rehabilitation at home and abroad, strengthen academic exchanges and cooperation, share experience and achievements, and promote the sound development of low vision rehabilitation in China, the Bureau of Medical Administration of Ministry of Health and the Rehabilitation Department of China Disabled

Persons' Federation started organizing the annual "International Low Vision Rehabilitation Forum" in 2009. China Visual Impairment Resource Centre (located in the Beijing Tongren Hospital) has been engaging in cultivation, training and standardized teaching of rehabilitation professionals, as well as scientific research and development. In 2011, the Centre started holding the "International Low Vision Rehabilitation Forum", which had been successfully held for ten sessions by 2019. Domestic experts on low vision and ophthalmologists interested in low vision rehabilitation have also actively participated in international low vision conferences, including the International Conference by the International Society for Low Vision Research and Rehabilitation. In addition, low vision has been increasingly valued by ophthalmic community, and the sessions for blindness prevention and low vision have been set at the annual meetings of the Congress of Chinese Ophthalmological Society, the Chinese Ophthalmologists Association, and many subspecialty societies, so as to facilitate the communication and study among the experts of low vision rehabilitation in China.

III. Low Vision Rehabilitation Plan

1. Low Vision or Visual Disability Rehabilitation Plan

In 1991, low vision rehabilitation was included into the *Outline on China's Disability Work in the 8ᵗʰ 5-year Plan period (1991-1995)*. Until the 13ᵗʰ 5-Year Plan period, CDPF has always been taking it as one of the key tasks. Through establishing the Low Vision Rehabilitation Department, training personnel, developing and supplying typoscopes, and publicizing knowledge, it has trained a large number of low vision rehabilitation personnel, and provided typoscopes for hundreds of thousands of patients with low vision. Moreover, it has also provided guarantee in aspects of institutions, personnel, professional knowledge and fund for low vision rehabilitation in China.

2. Attention to Low Vision Rehabilitation in Children and Adolescents

From 2009 to 2011, the central government offered special subsidies to support the "CDPF Rescue Rehabilitation Project for the Disabled Children in Poverty" throughout China. The "Rescue Rehabilitation Project for the Disabled Children Aged 0-6" was launched in multiple provinces (autonomous regions and municipalities directly under the central government), focusing on rehabilitation training and fitting of typoscopes for the visually disabled children. In 2013, Chinese government issued the *Notice on Issuing Technical Specifications for Children's Eye and Vision Care* (WBFSF [2013] No. 26), which explicitly stipulated the regular screening of eye diseases for the newborns. At present, China is gradually establishing a systematic system of eye care service, aiming to publicize the knowledge of prevention and treatment of eye diseases, timely discover the causal factors for disability, and carry out interventions as soon as possible to reduce the incidence of visual disabilities, save the economic loss, and lower the incidence of low vision in children.

IV. Achievements in low vision rehabilitation in China

1. Various Forms of Training for Low Vision Rehabilitation Personnel

The CDPF, National Health Commission of the People's Republic of China, and National Committee for the Prevention of Blindness organized annual training for backbone talents of low vision rehabilitation in all provinces (autonomous regions and municipalities directly under the central government). The provinces (autonomous regions and municipalitiesdirectly under the central government) have organized corresponding training classes based on the actual conditions and demands of each region. In addition, various societies and associations have also set up continuing educational training programs for ophthalmologists and rehabilitation doctors, aiming to improve the low vision screening and diagnosis capacity, strengthen the cooperation between ophthalmic institutions and low vision rehabilitation centers, and improve the quality of rehabilitation services through technical guidance.

2. Construction of the Low Vision Rehabilitation Network

As required in the *National Plan for the Prevention of Blindness (2012-2015)* (WYZF [2012] No. 52), each provincial rehabilitation center should establish its own "Low Vision Rehabilitation Center", and strengthen its ability building. In addition, a production and supply service network of low vision typoscopes should be established, aiming to improve the quality of life of low vision patients. The 13th 5-Year National Eye Health Plan (2016-2020) also required that the ophthalmology departments of tertiary general hospitals and eye hospitals should provide low-vision outpatient services, and all qualified hospitals should provide low vision rehabilitation services. As required, the cooperation and referral system between ophthalmic institutions and low vision rehabilitation centers should be established, the communication and cooperation between ophthalmic institutions and disease prevention and control institutions or eye disease prevention and treatment institutions, as well as low vision rehabilitation centers, should be strengthened. The cooperation mechanism integrating treatment, prevention and rehabilitation should be established.

In addition, the schools for the blind, where low vision children are concentrated, should carry out low vision classification teaching, visual function training, and training for parents. Moreover, they should also provide consulting services for the public. The trained parents should train their children on the visual function rehabilitation exercise and on the use of typoscopes at home.

3. Professional Fitting and Rehabilitation Training Supported by the Chinese Government

In the low vision/vision disability rehabilitation plan, CDPF required that the central and local finance departments should provide financial support for the fitting of typoscopes, and ensure the free provision of typoscope fitting and training. During the 11th 5-Year Plan period, free typoscopes were provided for 100,000 low vision children in poverty, and 30,000 parents of low vision children were trained. In addition, orientation and mobility training was also provided for 30,000 blind people [1]. During the 12th 5-Year Plan period, free typoscopes were provided for 500,000 low vision children, and 200,000 parents of low vision children were trained. In addition, orientation and mobility training and rehabilitation tools were provided for 500,000 blind people [2]. According to the *National Action Plan on Disability Prevention (2016—2020)* (GBF [2016] No. 66) launched by the General Office of the State Council, China will initially establish a relatively complete typoscope service network covering both the urban and rural areas, and establish a policy system that can ensure typoscope services for low vision patients in all local regions by 2020. It is expected that the service ability and situation for fitting typoscopes will be improved, and the fitting rate of the disabled with certificates and disabled children will reach over 80%.

4. Strong Support for The Research And Development of Typoscopes with Independent Property Rights

Typoscope fitting is one of the most direct and effective means to compensate for and improve the visual functions, quality of life, and social participation ability of low vision patients. During the 8th 5-Year Plan period, the assistive device service for the disabled was incorporated into the national economic and social development plan, which has made significant achievements so far. At the early stage of low vision rehabilitation in China, all typoscopes were imported. The first domestic typoscope was not developed until 1986. Under the policy support of the Ministry of   Health of People's Republic of China and CDPF, all provinces, autonomous region and municipalities directly under the central government guided and encouraged the enterprises, scientific research institutions, colleges and universities, and social organizations to participate in the development, research, production, distribution and prescription of typoscopes by fiscal, taxation, financial means, and distribution. Typoscopes of various brands and types have been gradually developed and marketed based the demands of low vision patients. At present, the work system of domestic typoscopes has been established, and the service system has been improved gradually.

5. Formation of A Coordinated Operation Mechanism Among All Departments

The health administrations at all levels have incorporated low vision rehabilitation into the scope of ophthalmology in hospitals and clarified the responsibilities of ophthalmologists in low vision rehabilitation and organized training for them. The education departments actively carried out work on low vision classification teaching and training for parents. CDPF also did important work on coordination, service, and publicity.

V. Summary

There is a large number of low vision patients in China. At present, progress on low vision rehabilitation has been made in China. Although there are many problems in the research of rehabilitation measures, it is predictable that there will be a complete and standardized evaluation and rehabilitation system developed and established, under the overall planning of the government and joint efforts of the whole society, especially the professionals, which can help low vision patients to improve their quality of life and participate in social life.

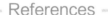

References

1. China Disabled Persons' Federation. The implementation plan of visual disability rehabilitation in the "11th 5-year plan" period [EB/OL].(2014-07-25)[2021-07-15]. http://2021old. cdpf. org. cn/ghjh/syfzgh/syw/201407/t20140725_357665. shtml.
2. China Disabled Persons' Federation. The development program of undertakings for the disabled in China in the "12th 5-year plan" period-supporting implementation plan iii : the implementation plan of visual disability rehabilitation in the "12th 5-year plan" period.[EB/OL].(2012-03-06)[2021-07-15]. http://2021old. cdpf. org. cn/ghjh/syfzgh/sew/201203/t20120306_78000. shtml.

Chapter X Promotion of Eye Health

Health promotion plays an important role in drawing the attention of sectors of society to health and gaining their support in making joint efforts to improve the health level of the whole society, so as to form a favorable social environment and atmosphere and achieve better health for all. Health promotion has become a preferred and core strategy for dealing with health issues in China. It was proposed in the report of the 19th National Congress of the Communist Party of China that we should promote the building of a Healthy China, indicating the Party and the government give high priority to people's health, and puting forward a higher requirement for the promotion of eye health.

I. Eye health promotion activities

In 1996, 12 ministries and commissions, including the national health administrations, the Ministry of Education, the Central Committee of the Communist Youth League of China, and CDPF, jointly issued a notice, in which, each June 6 was designated as the "National Eye Care Day"[1]. Until 2020, the "National Eye Care Day" has been organized 25 times in China for strengthening people's awareness of eye care and mobilizing all sectors of society to focus on eye health. The themes of the "National Eye Care Day" cover a variety of topics, including the vision of children and adolescents, eye health of the elderly, ocular trauma, cataract, childhood blindness, low vision, blinding trachoma, diabetic retinopathy, and myopia, etc. It intends to create a favorable atmosphere for active participation of the public in the prevention and treatment of eye diseases through providing education on eye health promotion, popularizing the knowledge about eye health, increasing the awareness of eye disease prevention, reducing the prevalence of different eye diseases, and increasing the awareness through designing theme and posters, and publicizing through radio, television, newspapers, and Internet, as well as other new media means.

In 2005, the March 15th Evening Party presented the case of "It's a pity that I cannot see the light ", and called for the public awareness of the harm of excessive oxygen inhalation and the prevention and treatment of retinopathy of prematurity. In recent years, with the training of medical personnel in the fields of the obstetrics, pediatrics and ophthalmology departments regarding the use of oxygen for emergency treatment of premature infants, as well as the prevention, diagnosis and treatment of retinopathy, establishing referral system between medical institutions for remote diagnosis and screening of retinopathy in premature infants, establishing committees for children care, organizing the training of medical care and health education for premature infants [2], promoting the suitable techniques and issuing the materials of health education, the incidence of retinopathy of prematurity and rate of severe symptom of retinopathy of prematurity have decreased year by year. In Shenzhen, for example, the incidence of retinopathy of prematurity and rate of severe symptom of retinopathy of prematurity were 14.64% and 6.52% in 2008, which decreased to 11.47% and 4.26% in 2013, indicating a significant drop compared with those in 1990s [3].

Health promotion on themed promotion days has been organized to promote the prevention of diabetic retinopathy, including the " World Diabetes Day " activities, health knowledge dissemination plans, daily health education activities, and screening activities at the communities, nursing homes, and centers for retired cadres jointly by the medical staff in ophthalmology and endocrinology departments. The hierarchical diagnosis and treatment service model between the primary medical and health institutions, endocrinology departments and ophthalmology departments was established. The awareness rate of diabetes and diabetic retinopathy has reached 76.7% [4] through the promotion of the guidelines for prevention and control of diabetes, as well as the knowledge about the prevention and treatment of its complications (including diabetic eye diseases) by publicity and education, free screening, consultation, science lectures, posters, and brochures through public media or the Internet. Such means have timely and effectively promoted the treatment of diabetic patients and increased the rate of early detection and early diagnosis of diabetic retinopathy.

The themed promotion activities of " Prevention of Myopia in Children and Adolescents " were organized throughout China. At present, all related departments (Ministry of Education, National Health Commission, General Administration of Sport, Ministry of Finance, Ministry of Human Resources and Social Security, State Administration for Market Regulation, National Press and Publication Administration, and National Radio and Television Administration), schools, medical and health institutions, families, and students have made joint efforts to take care of and protect the vision of children and adolescents. The whole society has been mobilized through extensive publicity and seminars, posters, parent meetings, parent letters, vision screening, and keeping visual health records. Children were encouraged to participate in the creation of comics on eye care and express their insights, so that they would take initiative in taking care of their eyes. The favorable atmosphere of " leadership by government, cooperation among sectors, guidance by experts, education in school, commitment in family " for protection of vision in children and adolescents has been created in the whole society.

The first World Glaucoma Week in China was on March 6, 2008, and by 2019, themed activities have been organized 11 times. The World Glaucoma Week, as a global initiative jointly initiated by the World Glaucoma Association and World Glaucoma Patient Association, intended to increase people's awareness of glaucoma, and reduce the undiagnosed rate of glaucoma from 50% to below 20% by 2020 [5]. In recent years, with the publicity through media, free consultation, glaucoma knowledge lectures, and patient experience sharing meetings by government departments, ophthalmologists and eye professionals, the detection rate of open-angle glaucoma has increased from 10% to 40% [6].

World Sight Day, the second Thursday of October every year, is a major publicity activity of "VISION 2020" initially held in 2000, and also a global medical public welfare action jointly established by the International Agency for the Prevention of Blindness, Lions Clubs International, and Orbis International, under the leadership of the WHO. Several voluntary agencies in China have organized publicity lectures, free consultation, vision screening, community education, and recycling of old glasses, to improve the public awareness of the blindness and visual impairment and to publicize blindness prevention and VISION 2020 initiative to the public.

II. Vigorous promotion of medical humanistic spirit

Ophthalmology is an important part of the clinical medical system. As for eye health, ophthalmology staff should not only deliver high-quality service on the clinical diagnosis and treatment of eye diseases but also pay attention to public health issues and work on the prevention of eye diseases and blindness. Through the vigorous promotion of the tradition of "Absolute Sincerity of Great Physicians, Heal the Wounded and Rescue the Dying", the Chinese government has encouraged eye care personnel, as well as primary medical and health workers, to provide eye care services for the people in poverty-stricken areas. In addition, eye care personnel have also participated in eye health promotion by means of radio, newspapers, television, and the Internet to enhance public awareness of the prevention and treatment of eye diseases and improve the work on prevention of eye diseases from the perspective of public health ophthalmology, which led to effectively improved eye disease prevention capacity and a better understanding of "VISION 2020: The Right to Sight". In order to recognize the outstanding contributions made by ophthalmology staff to the prevention of blindness, the Asia-Pacific Academy of Ophthalmology presented the "Outstanding Service in Prevention of Blindness

Awards " to 42 Chinese ophthalmology staff from 2005 to 2019. The Chinese Ophthalmological Society presented the " Outstanding Contribution in Prevention of Blindness Awards " to 6 ophthalmology staff in 2014 and 2016.

References

1. National Health Commission of People's Republic of China. National Eye-Care Day.[EB/OL].[2020-06-17]. http://www. nhc. gov. cn/jnr/qgayrjrjj/qgayr_lmtt. shtml.
2. CHEN Y, ZHU C, SHEN L, et al. Effectiveness evaluation of remote screening for retinopathy of prematurity [J]. Chinese journal of ocular fundus diseases, 2017, 33 (6): 633-634.
3. Shenzhen Cooperative Group for Retinopathy of Prematurity. The incidence of retinopathy of prematurity in Shenzhen during the past ten years [J]. Chinese journal of ocular fundus diseases, 2014, 30 (1): 12-16.
4. WANG D, DING X, HE M, et al. Use of eye care services among diabetic patients in urban and rural China [J]. Ophthalmology, 2010, 117 (9): 1755-1762.
5. National Health Commission of People's Republic of China. World Glaucoma Day.[EB/OL].(2014-03-04) [2020-06-17]. http://www. nhc. gov. cn/jnr/qgyjrjj/201403/238de4b376c74d699574f4bb3d7a489f. shtml.
6. LI H. Investigation on blindness rate of primary glaucoma in rural areas of Xiangtan [J]. Hunan medical journal, 1986 (3): 158.

Chapter XI   Development of Eye Banks in China

I. Overview

An eye bank refers to a medical organization or institution that is set in a medical institution for the purpose of obtaining, transferring, restoring, and handling cornea donated by people after death, as well as quality evaluation and distribution. The earliest eye banks in China included the Eye Bank of Beijing Tongren Hospital, Henan Eye Institute, Guangdong Branch Red Cross Society of China Corneal Donation Center, and Eye Bank of Shandong Eye Institute. In 1997, Eye Bank of Beijing Tongren Hospital, Eye Bank of EYE & ENT Hospital of Fudan University, and Eye Bank of Shandong Eye Institute officially joined the International Federation of Eye Banks as its formal members. The development of eye banks is closely related to the effective treatment of corneal blindness patients.

II. Current situation of and problems faced by eye banks in China

According to the survey, there are 78 eye banks in China. Compared with developed countries, the eye banks in China face the following issues: insufficient sources of cornea donors, and low-quality preprocessing of the cornea. The lack of donated corneas has become the fundamental cause affecting the development of eye banks in China and effective treatment of patients with treatable corneal blindness.

III. Progress

In view of the current development of and problems faced by eye banks in China, the Office of the National Committee for the Prevention of Blindness has promoted the related work since 2017 under the leadership of the Bureau of Medical Administration of National Health and Family Planning Commission:

(Ⅰ) Comprehensive survey on eye banks was carried out to better understand their current conditions. At present, there are 14 eye banks operating in China, which can process about 3,500 eyeballs and consume 2,800 corneas each year.

(Ⅱ) In 2018, the National Committee for the Prevention of Blindness established the Expert Committee for Management of Eye Banks, aiming to promote the development of eye banks in China, and improve the management and service quality of eye banks, involving the preparation of technical specifications for eye banks, establishment of eye bank management standards, promotion of the training for eye bank doctors and technicians, establishment of the national online donation information registration system, the improvement of public awareness of corneal donation, increase of people's awareness of cooperation in donation, and the establishment of an eye bank quality control system.

(Ⅲ) The specifications for the management of eye banks were developed. In order to standardize the construction and clarify the management requirements of eye banks, ensure the quality of donated cornea and medical safety, and safeguard the people's health, the Expert Committee for Management of Eye Banks of the National Committee for the Prevention of Blindness prepared *Eye Bank Management Specifications*, *Technical Guidelines for Operation of Eye Banks*, and *Eye Bank Quality Management and Control Indicators* under the guidance of national health administrations, all of which standardized the management and technical operation of eye banks in details, and the related quality control indicators were developed.

(Ⅳ) China's human cornea distribution and sharing system was established, which is used for whole-process management, equal distribution, and rational use of the donated corneas while complying with the medical needs and following the principles of fairness, impartiality, and openness. All corneas should be distributed and shared following the order stated in the waiting list of the transplant hospitals with eye banks, the waiting list of the transplant hospitals within the service area of eye banks, the waiting list at the level of provinces (autonomous regions, municipalities directly under the central government), and the national waiting list. The cornea distribution system is responsible for implementing the cornea distribution and sharing policy. All corneas must be distributed and shared through the cornea distribution system. No institution, organization, or individual is allowed to distribute any cornea without the use of the cornea distribution system. The system was piloted in 10 provinces (autonomous regions, municipalities directly under the central government) in October 2019.

Chapter XII Internationalization of Public Welfare Activities in Blindness Prevention in China

With the improvement in ophthalmic diagnosis and treatment capacity, public welfare activities for blindness prevention originating in China have also been promoted internationally.

In 2003, the National Committee for the Prevention of Blindness launched the " Sight Action " integrating epidemiological investigation, professional training, medical service, and health education based on the integration of national resources for blindness prevention. The medical teams have reached old revolutionary base areas, ethnic minorities concentrated areas, remote areas, poverty-stricken areas, and plateau areas and helped more than 40,000 cataract patients to recover their sight.

In 2008, the "Sight Action" was carried out outside China for the first time. Several medical teams were sent to Democratic People's Republic of Korea and Cambodia, as well as Mongolia, Laos, Vietnam, Bangladesh, and Pakistan in Asian-Pacific Region for public welfare activities. In 2010, the "Sight Action" was conducted in Africa and medical teams were sent to perform cataract surgeries in Zimbabwe, Malawi, Zambia, and Mozambique. In July 2012, the Chinese government announced at the Fifth Ministerial Conference of the Forum on China-Africa Cooperation new initiatives to deepen practical cooperation between China and Africa, including continued expansion of aid to Africa, such as " Sight Action" activities providing free treatment for cataract patients in Africa. At the opening ceremony of the Johannesburg Summit of the Forum on China-Africa Cooperation held in December 2015, Xi Jinping, general secretary of the Communist Party of China Central Committee, proposed " China-Africa Public Health Plan " as one of the " Ten Cooperation Plans for African Countries " to be implemented in the following three years.

In 2015, the National Health and Family Planning Commission issued the *Three-Year Implementation Plan for Promoting Health Exchanges and Cooperation Along the "Belt and Road"* (*2015-2017*)(GWBGJH [2015] No. 866), which clearly took the "Sight Action" as one of the important tasks of health development assistance. In order to further promote and implement the international health exchange and cooperation plan, provinces (autonomous regions, municipalities directly under the central government) sent medical teams to friendly countries to provide cataract surgery for local people. By far, China has sent medical teams to more than 40 countries, including Democratic People's Republic of Korea, Vietnam, Laos, Cambodia, Myanmar, Mongolia, Thailand, Bangladesh, Pakistan, Yemen, Bahamas, Zimbabwe, Malawi, Zambia, Mozambique, Burundi, Mauritania, Botswana, Jamaica, Antigua and Barbuda, Sri Lanka, Cameroon, Comorin, Republic of the Congo, Togo, Benin, Sudan, Senegal, Kazakhstan, Chad, Djibouti, Uzbekistan, Fiji, Tonga, Vanuatu, Samoa, Papua New Guinea, Micronesia, Cook Islands, Niue, Namibia, Sierra Leone. In more than ten of the above countries, the "Sight Action" has been conducted for multiple times, and tens of thousands of cataract patients have been treated.

In addition to providing of free cataract surgery and advanced ophthalmic surgical equipment and medicines for the local people, "Sight Action" has also performed vision screening for students, donated glasses, and carried out surgeries for patients with complicated fundus diseases and glaucoma. The medical teams have also held academic lectures and clinical teaching and established Ophthalmology Cooperation Centers in the relevant countries. In addition, they have also performed remote consultation on eye diseases through the Internet and adopted various forms of technical exchanges and cooperation. At the same time, great importance has been attached to talent training, and helped local doctors accept professional training in China.

The internationalization of China's public welfare activities in blindness prevention has brought light to the aided countries, fully demonstrating China's actions in building a community with a shared future for mankind, as well as the contributions to countries along the "Belt and Road". As an important force of China's diplomacy, the "Sight Action" has further promoted international health exchanges and cooperation.

Chapter XII Improvement of Independent Research and Development Ability

Ophthalmology is a comprehensive interdisciplinary discipline, and the diagnosis and treatment of eye diseases highly rely on ophthalmic equipment. Equipment quality, to a certain extent, determines the quality of diagnosis and treatment. With the development of modern high-technologies, ophthalmic equipment has been rapidly improved in clinical practicability, safety, intellectuality, and speed of update. They also played an important role in the prevention and treatment of eye diseases and guaranteeing medical quality.

I. Research & development and application of ophthalmic medical products and equipment

(I) Demand analysis of ophthalmic medical products

Ophthalmic medical products generally consist of ophthalmic equipment, ophthalmic consumables, ophthalmic drugs, and optic products. 70% of eye diseases are mainly treated through surgery, which highly relies on ophthalmic equipment. In 2017, the sales volume of ophthalmic medical devices and consumables reached USD 27.7 billion all over the world, accounting for 6.8% of the total sales of medical devices and consumables, making it the fifth largest market of medical devices. The sales volume is predicted to be USD 42.2 billion in 2024, with a compound growth rate of 6.2%, 5.6% higher than the overall sales volume of medical devices and consumables. The proportion of sales will increase to 7.1%. The size of the ophthalmic drug market in China has exceeded CNY 15 billion, and the development of innovative targeted drugs and formulations has strongly driven the growth of the market. In 2017, the size of the retail market of glasses reached CNY 73 billion, which is expected to further expand in 2020, reaching CNY 85 billion.

(II) General situation of development of domestic ophthalmic medical products

At present, the sales volume of the top 8 domestic enterprises of ophthalmic medical products accounts for 73.3% of the national market, of which, foreign brands account for nearly 50%. Domestic enterprises are generally small and inferior to foreign ones in technologies, high-end materials and the research and development fund, therefore, there is still great room for import substitution.

With the gradual improvement of medical insurance system and the progress of medical reform in China, the investment in blindness prevention in primary medical units has been increased year by year. Strengthening the research and development of ophthalmic treatment equipment suitable for primary level facilities to meet the eye care needs at primary level is of crucial importance for the overall development of national medical care and health. The retrieval of scientific research projects approved by the Ministry of Science and Technology showed that, during the periods of the 12th 5-Year Plan and the 13th 5-Year Plan, the research and development of small-scale, mobile medical service devices, high-value consumables, and innovative drugs for dealing with common eye diseases and frequently-occurring diseases were strongly supported, and CNY 90 million was invested in national research subjects.

In recent years, the ophthalmic resources have been significantly enriched, but they are still unevenly distributed. Especially in outlying poverty-stricken areas lack ophthalmic resources, there are no complete and sufficient basic ophthalmology services. Although activities such as "Sight Action" and free consultations have been organized in such areas by numerous medical institutions and social organizations, the traditional eye examination and treatment equipment cannot be widely used due to their large volume and difficulty in transportation. In recent years, several manufacturers have launched a variety of portable examination devices, such as portable optometers, slit lamps, and ophthalmoscopes, which can be used to increase the detection rate and accuracy of eye diseases, thus laying a foundation for effective treatment of the patients. In addition, portable treatment devices have also been developed, such as portable phaco emulsifiers and surgical microscopes.

In view of the complexity of eye diseases, a variety of ophthalmic equipment are required, including visual chart, slit lamp, direct/indirect ophthalmoscope, ophthalmotonometer, optometry unit, gonioscope, Three mirror contact lens, perimeter, ophthalmological A/B ultrasonic diagnostic apparatus, ultrasound biomicroscope (UBM), ophthalmometer, corneal endothelial cell counter, ophthalmic electrophysiological instrument, optical coherence tomography (OCT), corneal topographer, retinal fluorescence fundus imaging machine, YAG laser, photocoagulation laser, argon ion laser, surgical microscope, cataract phacoemulsifier, vitrectomy machine, and retinal cryoprobe.

Basically, common ophthalmic diagnostic facilities can be manufactured in China, and their market share has increased year by year. The ultrasound devices, OCT, and UBM have been exported to the overseas market. As for ophthalmic treatment equipment, doctors are paying more attention to their safety and stability, which have brought higher requirements for their technical and quality level. Domestic manufacturers are generally small and still inferior to foreign ones in technologies, high-end materials, and R&D funds. In particular, the devices for the treatment of cataract and myopia are still monopolized by foreign manufacturers.

The domestic ophthalmic drug market is highly concentrated: the three international giants occupy about 45.12% of the market share, and the leading domestic enterprises only occupy 14.03%. In the past five years, the leading domestic enterprises have made great progress in the development of innovative drugs for treating fundus neovascularization and xerophthalmia, with increasing market share.

In China, the market size of intraocular lens, the main consumables of cataract surgery, is about CNY 10 billion. In the past five years, domestic manufactures have made significant breakthroughs in soft (foldable) intraocular lens, with a market share of about 15%. The market of orthokeratology lens for controlling myopia in adolescents showed an explosive growth trend, from CNY 1.53 billion in 2014 to CNY 5.1 billion in 2018, increasing by about 30%. At present, the market share of domestic enterprises has reached about 20%.

Frame glasses are the most important devices for correcting refractive error. In European and American countries, frame glasses are classified as medical products in ophthalmic market; while in China, frame glasses belong to the consumer market due to historic reasons. The difference in market management departments made good frame glasses intermingled with bad ones in China. After years of development, the domestic market is still monopolized by foreign enter-prises. In recent years, domestic enterprises have made several technological breakthroughs in precise fitting and processing of lens, as well as customization of frames.

II. Research & development and application of remote ophthalmology and artificial intelligence (AI)

With the rapid development of information technology and the Internet, high-quality telemedicine services can be provided for the patients. In order to standardize the development of " Internet + " Healthcare, promote the application of telemedicine and provide more convenient medical services for the public, the National Health Commission and National Administration of Traditional Chinese Medicine launched the *Notice on Issuing the Measures for the*

Administration of Internet Diagnosis and Treatment and Other Two Documents (*Trial*) (GWYF [2018] No. 25), and prepared the *Measures for the Administration of Internet Diagnosis and Treatment* (*Trial*), *Measures for the Administration of Internet Hospitals* (*Trial*), and *Specifications for the Administration of Remote Medical Services* (*Trial*) on September 14, 2018, all of which were designed to further regulate Internet diagnosis and treatment and play the active role of telemedicine, to improve the efficiency of medical services.

Telemedicine has been rapidly popularized and promoted and played a very important role in balancing medical resources. By far all tertiary hospitals in China have set up teleophthalmology services, and all county-level hospitals in impoverished counties have been covered. On July 9, 2019, the National Health Commission reported at a press conference that tertiary hospitals dispatched more than 60,000 medical staff for the management of county-level hospitals in poverty-stricken counties and daily diagnosis and treatment by 2018. They admitted more than 30 million of outpatients and served more than 3 million discharged patients; in addition, they completed more than 500,000 operations. Based on their dissemination, assistance, and guidance, 5,900 clinical specialties were established in county-level hospitals, and more than 38,000 new technologies and projects were implemented. More than 400 county-level hospitals in impoverished counties were promoted to secondary hospitals, and 30 to tertiary hospitals. The high-quality medical services of tertiary hospitals helped to significantly improve the service capacity and management level of hospitals in impoverished counties.

Ophthalmology generally adopts imaging as the main auxiliary diagnostic means, and it is the most suitable discipline for telemedicine by virtue of its great advantages. Telemedicine will help to distribute high-quality medical resources to county-level hospitals, and solve the problem of uneven distribution of ophthalmic resources. Previous studies showed that ophthalmic telemedicine could be more cost-effective in the screening of chronic eye diseases, such as diabetic retinopathy and glaucoma [1]. Several ophthalmic telemedicine systems have been developed in China, with great performance. The collaborative model between tertiary hospitals and primary hospitals based on remote eye consultation centers has provided an effective and convenient means for screening and diagnosis of eye diseases [2].

The rapid development of AI has also brought about new breakthroughs in auxiliary ophthalmic diagnosis and treatment and disease prediction. On November 15, 2017, the Ministry of Science and Technology held the " Kick-Off Meeting for the New Generation Artificial Intelligence Development Plan and Major Science and Technology Projects " , which introduced the organization and promotion mechanism for the implementation of the "New Generation Artificial Intelligence Development Plan", and announced the establishment of the Promotion Office of the " New Generation Artificial Intelligence Development Plan " . Moreover, it introduced the preliminary preparations for the implementation of the " New Generation Artificial Intelligence Development Plan " and emphasized the establishment of an open and collaborative AI technology innovation system for implementation of the Plan. Finally, it also announced a list of the earliest national new-generation AI open innovation platforms, including the platforms for medical imaging.

In December 2017, National Health and Family Planning Commission issued the *Technical Guidelines for Application of Hospital Informatization* (GWBGHH [2017] No. 1232), which put forward the technical requirements for specific application of AI in health and medical services, medical intelligent applications and hospital intelligent management. In April 2018, the National Health Commission issued the *Standards and Norms for Hospital Informatization* (*Trial*) (GWBGHF [2018] No. 4), which put forward specific requirements for AI applications in hospitals, such as prediction of disease risks, medical imaging assisted diagnosis, clinical assisted diagnosis and treatment, intelligent health management, hospital intelligent management, and virtual assistants.

At present, AI ophthalmic imaging has been applied in the diagnosis of a variety of blinding eye diseases, including cataract, glaucoma, diabetic retinopathy, and age-related macular degeneration. Taking diabetic retinopathy as an example, the data released by the International Diabetes Federation (IDF) in 2018 showed that about 500 million Chinese people had prediabetes, about 110 million had diabetes, and about 30 million had diabetic retinopathy [3]. AI can screen and diagnose diabetic retinopathy at the early stage with a promising accuracy. In recent years, a variety of enterprises and research institutions have carried out the related research, and enterprises have developed intelligent algorithms for quality assessment of fundus images, severity classification of diabetic retinopathy, and detection of lesion location, which can automatically generate structured screening reports, and thus providing referral recommendations for the patients. The statistics on glaucoma performed in 2011 showed that its prevalence was 2.6%, with the blindness rate of 30%, in Chinese people over 40. The direct cost of treatment of all patients would be USD 15-18 billion [4,5]. At present, a deep learning algorithm developed by a domestic research team for automatic detection of glaucomatous optic nerve damage based on fundus images [6] has realized the visualization of AI recognition process. OPTOMERTY TIMES did a special report on it as " the first multi-center study from the real world in China " . In addition, the team has also developed the first glaucoma visual screening product in China in cooperation with Internet company. At present, AI can be used to diagnose common blinding eye diseases and predict the development of myopia in children [7].

At the 9th Session of Focus Group on Artificial Intelligence for Health [①] (FG AI4H) held in May 2020, two application standards and technical requirements about " AI Imaging Tech-

---

① Focus Group on Artificial Intelligence for Health was co-founded by WHO and International Telecommunication Union, committing to the standard pre-research of AI in health care.

nology in Fundus Disease Screening" submitted by the team from Beijing were adopted by the FG AI4H[8,9], indicating that AI image screening for fundus diseases in China has been used as an international standard for AI in health and medical care. In the future, it will be the recommended standard in AI medical care recognized by the WHO and International Telecommunication Union, for reference by drug regulatory agencies and related medical enterprises in various countries. It is believed that AI will bring comprehensive innovation from screening to diagnosis in the near future with the continuous development of AI and further improvement of the related policies, thus introducing new vitality to ophthalmology.

References

1. SHARAFELDIN N, KAWAGUCHI A, SUNDARAM A, et al. Review of economic evaluations of teleophthalmology as a screening strategy for chronic eye disease in adults [J]. Br J Ophthalmol, 2018, 102 (11): 1485-1491.
2. ZHANG L, XU J, CAO K, et al. The role of teleophthalmology consulting in improving glaucoma diagnosis in population [J]. Chin j ophthalmol med (electronic edition), 2019, 9 (4): 206-211.
3. International Diabetes Federation. IDF Diabetes Atlas.[EB/OL].[2020-06-02]. http://www. diabetesatlas. org/.
4. REIN D, ZHANG P, WIRTH K, et al. The economic burden of major adult visual disorders in the United States [J]. Archives of ophthalmology, 2006, 124 (12): 1754-1760.
5. LIANG Y, FRIEDMAN D, ZHOU Q, et al. Prevalence of primary open angle glaucoma in a rural adult Chinese population: the Handan eye study [J]. Investigative ophthalmology & visual science, 2011, 52 (11): 8250-8257.
6. LIU H, LI L, WORMSTONE I, et al. Development and validation of a deep learning system to detect glaucomatous optic neuropathy using fundus photographs [J]. JAMA ophthalmology, 2019, 137 (12): 1353-1360.
7. LIN H, LONG E, DING X, et al. Prediction of myopia development among Chinese school-aged children using refraction data from electronic medical records: A retrospective, multicentre machine learning study [J]. Plos med, 2018, 15 (11): 167-175.
8. WU J, ZHU Y, ZHANG Y, et al. Evaluation method and index of artificial intelligence glaucoma assisted screening system based on fundus image [Z]. ITU-T Focus Group on AI for Health, International Telecommunication Union. 2020.
9. WU J, ZHU Y, ZHANG Y, et al. Data set construction and annotation of artificial intelligence assisted screening system based on fundus image [Z]. ITU-T Focus Group on AI for Health, International Telecommunication Union. 2020.

Chapter XIV   Eye Health Challenges in China

The epidemiological study on eye diseases is one of the basic tasks for the prevention and treatment of blindness. In recent years, several large-scale epidemiological studies have been completed in China, such as the The Liwan Eye Study, The Kailuan Eye Study, The Beijing Eye Study, and The Handan Eye Study [1-4], which have provided a wealth of reliable evidence for basic understanding of current eye health in China. The data obtained from above-mentioned epidemiological studies and those on burden of eye diseases completed in recent years showed that the burden of eye health was basically stable with slight changes [5].

I. Refractive error and cataract ranked top 2 in terms of disease burden

Specifically, from 1990 to 2020 [5], refractive error has always been the leading cause of ocular disease burden and the main cause of vision impairment in all age groups, with its age-standardized prevalence of refractive error much higher than other eye diseases. Cataracts ranked the second (Fig.14-1, Fig. 14-2). Refractive error and cataracts are the most important causes of ocular disease burden in China.

II. The prevalence steadily declined, but the number affected has increased

From the prevalence point of view, prevalence in each age group remained basically stable, ranking as follows: refractive error first and cataracts ranked second. At the same time, we can see a clear trend: with the population aging, although the age-standardized prevalence of refractive error and cataract did not increased significantly from 1990 to 2020, basically remaining stable, but due to the total population growth and population aging, the number of patients affected by refractive error and cataract greatly increased.

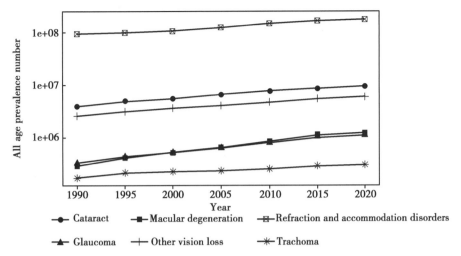

Fig.14-1 The number of patients with major eye diseases in China from 1990 to 2020

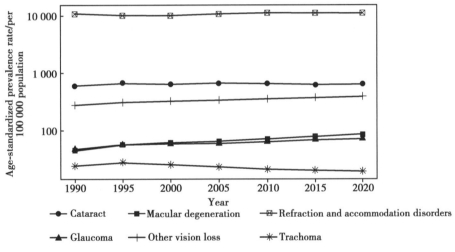

Fig.14-2 The age-standardized prevalence of major eye diseases in China from 1990 to 2020

III. The maculopathy is on the rise

It is also worth noting that the quantity of patients with glaucoma was greater than that of patients with macular degeneration before 2005, but after 2005, the number of patients with macular degeneration increased year by year and surpassed that of the patients with glaucoma. In addition, the age-standardized prevalence of glaucoma was surpassed by that of maculopathy in 2000. The maculopathy, a fundus disease, is often associated with people's living standards and lifestyles. Both the government and the public should attach importance to the prevention and control of fundus diseases.

IV. The burden of eye disease has increased the most among the middle-aged and elderly population

From 1990 to 2015, both the number of patients with eye diseases and years lived with disability in population aged 0-14 decreased significantly (Fig.14-3). In population aged 15 and above, especially in population aged 50 and above, the two indicators increased significantly.

In 1990, the prevalence of glaucoma in population aged 50 and above ranked the fourth, and that of macular degeneration ranked the fifth. In 2015, the prevalence of macular degeneration in population aged 50 and above ranked the fourth, and that of glaucoma fell to the fifth.

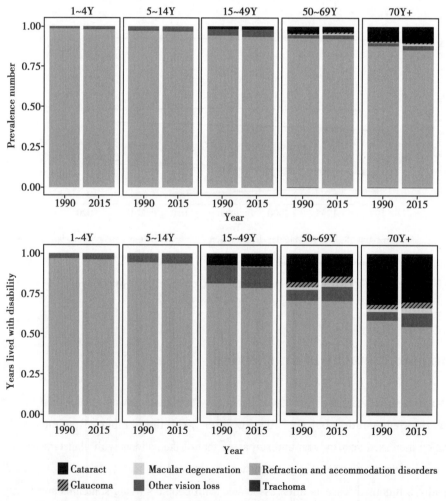

Fig.14-3 The quantity of patients with eye diseases and years lived with disability in all age groups in China from 1990 to 2015

In conclusion, the greatest challenge in eye health is the increase in and aging of population in China. In 2019, the population over 60 reached 253.88 million, accounting for 18.1% of the overall population, and the population of the aged is persistently increasing, indicating the continuous increase in the number of patients with age-related eye diseases, including refractive error and cataract, both of which have become the main cause of eye disease burden in China. In addition, the common blinding eye diseases, including the fundus diseases such as glaucoma and maculopathy, are all age-related eye diseases. As compared with the young, the prevalence of such diseases is usually higher in the aged. They are the challenges and key focus in eye health work in China in the future.

References

1. YAN Y, WANG Y, YANG Y, et al. Ten-year progression of myopic maculopathy: the Beijing eye study 2001-2011 [J]. Ophthalmology, 2018, 125 (8): 1253-1263.
2. WANG L, ZHAO Y, HAN X, et al. Five-year visual outcome among people with correctable visual impairment: the Liwan eye study [J]. Clin exp ophthalmol, 2018, 46 (5): 462-467.
3. WANG Q, WANG Y, WU S, et al. Ocular axial length and diabetic retinopathy: the Kailuan eye study [J]. Invest ophthalmol vis sci, 2019, 60 (10): 3689-3695.
4. CAO K, HAO J, ZHANG Y, et al. Design, methodology, and preliminary results of the follow-up of a population-based cohort study in rural area of northern China: Handan eye study [J]. Chin med j (engl), 2019, 132 (18): 2157-2167.
5. WANG B, CONGDON N, BOURNE R, et al. Burden of vision loss associated with eye disease in China 1990-2020: findings from the Global Burden of Disease Study 2015 [J]. Br j ophthalmol, 2018, 102 (2): 220-224.

Afterword

With the changes in lifestyle, social development, and population aging, great changes have taken place in the spectrum of eye diseases in China, therefore, eye health shall be incorporated in general health, and the eye health plan shall be prepared according to the "Outline of the Healthy China 2030". The 14th 5-Year Eye Health Plan should be prepared based on national realities, shifting the focus from common blinding eye diseases to major blinding eye diseases such as keratopathy, glaucoma, metabolism-related eye diseases, and age-related eye diseases. Actions should be taken to change the regional imbalance in the allocation of ophthalmic resources, promote balanced development, and transfer the focus from treatment to prevention of blinding eye diseases. In addition, particular attention should be paid to the application of techniques for the prevention and treatment of blinding eye diseases in primary hospitals, the strengthening of the construction of primary ophthalmology and ophthalmic teams, and improvement of the construction of the three-tier blindness prevention system. At the same time, relying on health-promotion-driven poverty alleviation projects such as the Standardized Training to Elevate Eyecare in rural China, the ophthalmology service capacity building should be combined with the national poverty alleviation work to promote the progress in building Healthy China through health-promotion-driven poverty alleviation.

The evaluation indicators of cataract surgery should be determined according to national realities, and the indications should be adjusted according to the level of social and economic development. The cataract surgery should be evaluated based on not only the quantity, but more importantly the quality, and the attention should be paid to the new indicator proposed by WHO, the effective coverage of cataract surgery. The national implementation plan for the prevention and control of myopia should be resolutely implemented to realize the national goal of the prevention and control of myopia in children and adolescents while keeping close attention to the new indicator proposed by WHO, the effective coverage of refractive error.

In addition, as for commonly used ophthalmic equipment and technologies, localization should be vigorously promoted, to reduce the high dependence on imported equipment and technologies and to make breakthroughs in common and key technologies. All institutions involved should continue to promote the training and promotion of appropriate technologies for preventable and controllable blinding eye diseases, so as to reduce the incidence and increase the control effect. When the technologies are well-developed, the screening of eye diseases based on AI should be promoted, to realize early detection and early treatment of blinding eye diseases. If the national economic conditions permit, considering that the number of patients with eye diseases caused by systemic diseases is on the rise, the screening of common blinding eye diseases should be incorporated into the chronic disease management system. Myopia in children and adolescents has become the main cause of visual impairment in China. Health education should be carried out to enhance the understanding of the basic knowledge for prevention and treatment of eye diseases, increase the awareness rate, and enhance the awareness of prevention and control of blinding eye diseases among the public. Science popularization should be incorporated into the national eye health plans and science popularization of health in China.

Under the leadership of the National Health Commission, ophthalmic communities should form two cooperation circles. Internationally, they should work closely with the World Health Organization, the International Agency for the Prevention of Blindness, the International Council of Ophthalmology, and other institutions to share the progress in China's eye health work with the world. Domestically, cooperation with various societies such as the Chinese Preventive Medicine Association and the Chinese Ophthalmological Society should be established. With the support of domestic academic teams and medical units, ophthalmic communities should work together for improved eye health work in China.

Acknowledgements

The Party and government have always been attaching great importance to eye health work. It is under the leadership and support of the national health departments and under the guidance of eye health policy that China's eye health work has made great progress. Here, a special " thank you " goes to the National Health Commission for its long-term guidance on the prevention of blindness and eye health, as well as the guidance for the preparation and compilation of the White Paper. In addition, our gratitude goes to the World Health Organization for its long-term support to China's blindness prevention and eye health work, as well as its technical guidance for work on trachoma prevention and control, the implementation of the third phase of " Sight First China Action" , and personnel training, etc. In addition, the International Agency for the Prevention of Blindness has provided long-term support for blindness prevention work in China and made important contributions to the promotion of appropriate technologies in China. Last but not least, the authors would like to express sincere thanks to the eye health workers nationwide for their joint efforts in promoting eye health in China and for their strong support in the process of preparing this White Paper.